Bacteriology Research Developments

GERMS AND TISSUES:
FRANK MACFARLANE BURNET,
PETER BRIAN MEDAWAR,
AND THE IMMUNOLOGICAL
CONJUNCTURE

BACTERIOLOGY RESEARCH DEVELOPMENTS

Handbook on Cyanobacteria: Biochemistry, Biotechnology and Applications
Percy M. Gault and Harris J. Marler (Editors)
2009. 978-1-60741-092-8

Methicillin-Resistant Staphylococcus Aureus (MRSA): Etiology, At-Risk Populations and Treatment
Charles L. Kolendi (Editor)
2009. 978-1-60741-398-1

Biodegradation of Cellulose Fibers
Barbara Simončič, Brigita Tomšič, Boris Orel and Ivan Jerman
2010. 978-1-61668-154-8

Germs and Tissues: Frank Macfarlane Burnet, Peter Brian Medawar, and the Immunological Conjuncture
Hyung Wook Park
2010. 978-1-61668-411-2

Bacteriology Research Developments

GERMS AND TISSUES: FRANK MACFARLANE BURNET, PETER BRIAN MEDAWAR, AND THE IMMUNOLOGICAL CONJUNCTURE

HYUNG WOOK PARK

Nova Science Publishers, Inc.
New York

Copyright © 2010 by Nova Science Publishers, Inc.

All rights reserved. No part of this book may be reproduced, stored in a retrieval system or transmitted in any form or by any means: electronic, electrostatic, magnetic, tape, mechanical photocopying, recording or otherwise without the written permission of the Publisher.

For permission to use material from this book please contact us:
Telephone 631-231-7269; Fax 631-231-8175
Web Site: http://www.novapublishers.com

NOTICE TO THE READER

The Publisher has taken reasonable care in the preparation of this book, but makes no expressed or implied warranty of any kind and assumes no responsibility for any errors or omissions. No liability is assumed for incidental or consequential damages in connection with or arising out of information contained in this book. The Publisher shall not be liable for any special, consequential, or exemplary damages resulting, in whole or in part, from the readers' use of, or reliance upon, this material.

Independent verification should be sought for any data, advice or recommendations contained in this book. In addition, no responsibility is assumed by the publisher for any injury and/or damage to persons or property arising from any methods, products, instructions, ideas or otherwise contained in this publication.

This publication is designed to provide accurate and authoritative information with regard to the subject matter covered herein. It is sold with the clear understanding that the Publisher is not engaged in rendering legal or any other professional services. If legal or any other expert assistance is required, the services of a competent person should be sought. FROM A DECLARATION OF PARTICIPANTS JOINTLY ADOPTED BY A COMMITTEE OF THE AMERICAN BAR ASSOCIATION AND A COMMITTEE OF PUBLISHERS.

LIBRARY OF CONGRESS CATALOGING-IN-PUBLICATION DATA

Available upon Request
ISBN: 978-1-61668-411-2

Published by Nova Science Publishers, Inc. ✢ New York

CONTENTS

Preface		vii
Chapter 1	Introduction	1
Chapter 2	Age, Microbes, and the Causes of Infectious Disease in Frank Macfarlane Burnet' Research	5
Chapter 3	Growth, Aging, and Tissue Transplantation in Peter Brian Medawar's Research	23
Chapter 4	Conclusion	45
References		47
Index		55

PREFACE

The Nobel Prize in Physiology and Medicine in 1960 was awarded to two renowned scientists in Australia and Britain, Frank Macfarlane Burnet and Peter Brian Medawar. Many historical accounts have described Burnet's theoretical prediction of immunological "tolerance" and its experimental confirmation by Medawar as a momentous achievement in immunology. In this monograph, I illuminate the two scientists' research pathways, especially their different ways of approaching the immunological changes of the host organism during embryogenesis and fetal development. Burnet was trained in medicine and studied infectious disease. By investigating the ecological and evolutionary relationship between the host and the pathogen, particularly the changing outcome of infection in accordance with the host's age, he arrived at the conclusion that immunological "self" is determined during developmental periods and any entities that entered the host during these periods will be permanently "tolerated." In contrast, Medawar received no formal medical education and never studied infectious disease. However, he built his expertise in tissue transplantation by participating in a research project on treating burned patients through skin grafting during World War II. Simultaneously, he developed an evolutionary theory of aging under the influence of his contemporary British scientists, such as R. A. Fisher, D'Arcy Thompson, and Julian Huxley. His success in demonstrating the tolerance phenomenon was derived from combining his knowledge and expertise in these two domains, tissue transplantation and evolutionary study of aging. This monograph will argue that while both Burnet and Medawar came to focus on the growing organism's changing state with its age in their research on immunological "self" and "tolerance," they did so in very distinctive ways. Burnet created his theory through his study of infectious disease, while Medawar designed and conducted his experiment through his aging theory and expertise in tissue transplantation. By analyzing these differences, I will show that the discovery of tolerance was not an example of applying the hypothetico-deductive method—initiated by Burnet's theory and Medawar's subsequent confirmation of it—but the product of an accidental conjuncture of multiple traditions and methodologies in biomedicine.

This monograph is a modified version of a chapter in Annette W. Barton (ed.), Host-pathogen interactions: genetics, immunology, and physiology. Hauppauge: Nova Science; 2010. The part on Frank Macfarlane Burnet stems from my previous paper, Hyung Wook Park, Germs, hosts, and the origin of Frank Macfarlane Burnet's theory of "self" and "tolerance," 1936-1949. *J Hist Med All Sci* 2006;61:492-534.

Chapter 1

INTRODUCTION

Frank Macfarlane Burnet (1899-1985) and Peter Brian Medawar (1915-1987) shared the Nobel Prize in Physiology and Medicine in 1960 for their significant contribution to immunology. In his *Production of Antibodies* (1949), Burnet proposed a theory which predicted that any entity that existed in an organism's body during its embryonic and fetal period would be regarded as its "self" and be permanently "tolerated" [1]. In 1953, Medawar conducted a tissue transplantation experiment relevant to this prediction, showing that genetically distinct cells implanted into a mouse fetus would not only be perpetually tolerated but also make the host body accept any tissues from the original donor strain after the end of its growth phase [2]. Many later researchers and historians of science have regarded these works of Burnet and Medawar as one of the most significant accomplishments in modern immunology [3-20]. For some of them, Burnet's and Medawar's contribution led to the rise of biological perspectives in immunology that had been dominated by chemical researchers until the mid-twentieth century [7-10]. Burnet and Medawar have also been mentioned as creators of conceptual, linguistic, and social bridges connecting laboratory scientists and clinicians involved in immunological research and practice [11].

Despite this contribution that they made together, Burnet and Medawar had little in common in terms of nationality, physical location, education, and major study topics. Burnet was an Australian scientist working at the Walter and Eliza Hall Institute in Melbourne, while Medawar was Professor of Zoology at University College London in England. Their difference in training and primary research subject was as wide as the physical distance between Melbourne and London. Burnet was trained in medicine and was primarily interested in infectious disease, whereas Medawar did not receive any formal medical education and never investigated infectious disease. He studied basic biology during his education in Magdalen College and the Department of Zoology at the University of Oxford, and later adopted tissue transplantation as his main research methodology and study subject. How, then, did these differences influence their research in immunology? Can we find any meaningful distinctions in the two scientists' approaches and standpoints that reflect their training, research experience, methodology, and direction of research?

The significance of these differences becomes more striking by the fact that there was little interaction between the two scientists. In his autobiography, Burnet wrote that he kept meeting with Medawar after 1946, mostly "over sandwiches and beer at the local pub" during his occasional visits to England [21]. However, Medawar's autobiography does not say anything about their meetings and discussions. Moreover, their archival collections do not show much evidence that Burnet and Medawar interacted with each other through intimate contact and scholarly discussion. During the 1940s and 1950s, they exchanged few letters concerning their scientific research, and never tried to initiate or pursue a cooperative project. Indeed, the major means of their academic communication was limited to their publications.

Despite their infrequent academic interactions, it is often easy to think that their achievement resulted from a set of close cooperative research following the hypothetico-deductive method. A simplistic version of the story can be like the following: Burnet provided a hypothesis on the formation of immune "self" and "tolerance," which was subsequently tested and proved by his colleague, Medawar. Although partially true, this kind of story does not properly reflect the complex process of actual scientific research as well as the difference between the two scientists. Some people may wonder whether Medawar's reading of Burnet's publications was enough for him to design and implement an experiment confirming Burnet's idea. But historians of science have already shown that published materials may not be sufficient in scientific communication and initiation of collaborative research like the one that was allegedly pursued by Burnet and Medawar [22]. While closer and even personal interaction was often necessary for two or more scientists trained in different fields to propose and confirm a thesis in a cooperative manner, the geographic and academic distance between Burnet and Medawar were just too wide. In fact, Medawar himself criticized simplistic accounts about Burnet's and his achievement. He disliked "a conventional theory" which postulated that "Burnet predicted on theoretical grounds that tolerance must exist as an empirical phenomenon, whereupon Medawar and his friends showed it did" [16].

In retrospect, this misleading view of the relationship between Burnet and Medawar stems from the two scientists' highest honor, the Nobel Prize, which was awarded to them because of Burnet's theoretical prediction and Medawar's experimental confirmation of it. But I think that the fact that they shared the Nobel Prize for such a reason can be misleading. Since the Prize is just an institutionalized means of acknowledging scientists' contributions, it does not reveal a deeper and more complex aspect of the relationship among the co-winners. In this sense, it is remarkable that both Burnet and Medawar wanted to share the Prized with different people. Burnet hoped that it would have been better if the Prize had been jointly awarded to Burnet and the Danish scientist Niels Jerne, whereas Medawar wished that he would have shared the Prize with the coauthors of the landmark 1953 paper, Rupert Billingham and Leslie Brent [6, 23].

Reflecting these problems in the conventional stories about Burnet and Medawar, this monograph provides an alternative explanation by using a comparative analysis. I show that Burnet's and Medawar's achievements did not result from a coherent hypothetico-deductive method or a close collaboration between the two scientists. I argue that their success stemmed from a contingent *conjuncture* of various fields and subdisciplines in biology and medicine, including medical virology, epidemiology, research on cytoplasmic inheritance, tissue transplantation, and mathematical and theoretical study of growth and aging. Although there were some interactions between the two scholars, they maintained their unique research style and approaches which originated from the distinct institutional environment and training. I will point out that Burnet's medical education and research on viruses and infectious disease became a basis of his theoretical proposal of "self" and "tolerance" while Medawar's mathematical and theoretical study of growth and aging was combined with his expertise in tissue transplantation in his successful experiment on "actively acquired tolerance."

This monograph also analyzes the two scientists' similarities as well as differences to explain how their work achieved such a "conjuncture." "Conjuncture" is a term used by historian and philosopher of life science Hans-Jörg Rheinberger to designate a situation in which two or more seemingly unrelated lines of research can meet and produce an unexpected result [24]. I think that Rheinberger's term can help us understand the relationship between Burnet and Medawar. Even though they worked in very distinctive ways and were educated in highly different environments, they appreciated, in a relatively independent manner, the importance of age in embryonic and fetal development and conceived the idea that immunological identity was formed during growth phases. It is also significant that they simultaneously came to employ cytoplasmic inheritance theories in conceptualizing this idea, although their ways of using them were highly different. Furthermore, both Burnet and Medawar tried to prove their idea of immunological identity formation through their experiments, although only Medawar was successful in this attempt.

In describing these similarities and differences, I challenge what several historical works on Burnet and Medawar imply, namely, the idea that Burnet was an ingenious theoretician and "biological thinker" [9, 10, 25] while Medawar was an experimentalist. Admittedly, these designations were partially right, because Burnet's genius in theory-making and biological perspectives made a substantial contribution to immunology. But Medawar's capacity as a theoretician has attracted less attention than it deserves. In most historical literature dealing with immunological "tolerance," Medawar is mentioned only as a scientist who conducted the first experiment demonstrating tolerance phenomenon. Certainly, this problem reflects the two scientists' alleged respective roles in the conceptualization of "self" and experimental induction of "tolerance," which led the two scholars to share the Nobel Prize. But I point out that both scholars were great theoretician and ingenious experimentalist at the same time, although their theories and experiments represented their differences in educational background, approach, and research priority. Given these distinct trajectories and similar points, I will show, both Burnet and Medawar ultimately contributed to the birth of the concept of "self" and "tolerance" which was immensely influential upon the later developments in immunology.

Chapter 2

AGE, MICROBES, AND THE CAUSES OF INFECTIOUS DISEASE IN FRANK MACFARLANE BURNET' RESEARCH

Born in Traralgon, Australia, Frank Macfarlane Burnet completed his medical education in 1924 at the University of Melbourne. He then went to England and finished his Ph.D. training in 1927 at the University of London through his study of *Salmonella* and bacteriophages. During his years at London, Burnet was substantially influenced by his academic advisors, J. C. G. Ledingham and J. A. Arkwright. As historian of science Olga Amsterdamska has shown, Ledingham and Arkwright were renowned medical researchers who were interested in the new problems concerning microbes and infectious disease [26]. While Robert Koch, the German bacteriologist and a strong advocate of the germ theory of disease, postulated the invariability of microbes and their straightforward causal relation to infectious diseases, Ledingham and Arkwright studied the variability of microbes and "healthy carriers" whose existence raised questions on the assumptions of Koch and other champions of early germ theories. Whereas these doctors often thought that the patient's body was just a passive medium in which a specific germ caused a particular disease, Burnet's advisors held that germs could actively change their characteristics and the host body could also be a key factor of disease causation. For Ledingham and Arkwright, the study of healthy carriers raised issues supporting their view. Why did some people fail to develop any symptoms after being infected with a specific pathological agent? Whereas both the host and the pathogen could be involved in this phenomenon, Ledingham and Arkwright focused on the host in their renowned monograph,

The Carrier Problem in Infectious Disease (1912). In this book, they suggested that the nonsymptomatic "carrier" states might pertain to the host body's immune system [27]. As we will see, Burnet's later research showed that he absorbed these scholars' ideas and became deeply concerned about the host body's role in the development of infectious disease.

In retrospect, Burnet's advisors, as well as Burnet himself after finishing graduate education, were departing from the paradigm of infectious disease that had been established in the late nineteenth century by Koch, Louis Pasteur, and other scholars. While the traditional Western medicine examined diverse factors regarding patients' constitution and environments as causes of disease—such as patients' gender, age, temper, humoral balance, or bad air—the germ theory of disease promoted by Koch and others claimed that a specific type of germs was the most important, if not the only, cause of a certain disease [28]. Burnet spent his time in England where the influence of this new medical thinking was less enthusiastically received than other European countries, as medical historian Michael Worboys has shown [29]. In this country, Burnet's advisors were two of the most prominent British scientists who were illuminating certain aspects of microbial infection which had not been intensively discussed by Koch and Pasteur.

After returning to Australia in 1927 as an assistant director of the Walter and Eliza Hall Institute, Burnet undertook a research project on a problem that could be solved by the perspectives he acquired in England. In 1928, Charles Kellaway, director of the Hall Institute, ordered Burnet to investigate the "Bundaberg tragedy," a severe incident involving the death of twelve children among the twenty-one who had been inoculated with a diphtheria vaccine at Bundaberg, Queensland [6]. After a laboratory test, Burnet quickly found an apparent problem—the vaccine was contaminated with a strain of *Staphylococcus*. But the cause of the tragedy was not immediately clear, because the strain of *Staphylococcus* was one that was commonly found in normal human skin. How, then, did such a usual germ bring about the highly tragic consequence at Bundaberg? He thought that the real cause of the incident could be found in the fact that the germ, which was neutral by itself in its normal habitat, was suddenly introduced underneath the skin in a large number through vaccination. This indicated that the presence of the germ, which was considered a crucial factor by Koch, was not enough to cause a fatality. Two other factors, namely, the germ's location and its number, were important as well. Even a perfectly benign microbe in its natural condition could severely harm the host if it were to be placed in an unnatural environment and in an excessive number.

The issue that this research raised was the importance of *natural balance*, which, if disturbed artificially, could lead to disease and death. As will be shown in this section, Burnet was deeply interested in this subject and returned to it whenever he encountered problems concerning infectious diseases and immunity. His theorization of immunological "self" and "tolerance" was also indebted to his thoughts on this issue.

Burnet's thinking on the nature of bacteriophages was also closely related to his idea on natural state and balance. Burnet kept studying bacteriophages after finishing his Ph.D. dissertation, and proposed an idea revealing his strong conviction about ecological equilibrium in his papers published during the early 1930s. In these writings, Burnet supported the French-Canadian microbiologist Félix d'Herelle's argument that the bacteriophage was a virus infecting bacteria rather than the Belgian immunologist Jules Bordet's claim that it was merely a microbial enzyme. To Burnet, a key proof that d'Herelle was right came from the phenomenon of lysogeny, which he interpreted as a "symbiosis" between bacteria and phages [30, 31]. Through his own experimental research, Burnet, like d'Herelle, arrived at his conclusion that bacteria and phages were distinct organisms that had lived together during their long evolutionary process, which enabled their symbiosis in the form of lysogeny. Remarkably, Burnet also accounted for the carrier state of humans' infectious disease as a kind of symbiosis between people and microbes [32, 33]. For him, both lysogeny and carrier state were examples of harmonious coexistence and balance between the host and the parasite, which could be frequently observed in nature.

Burnet found another example of this coexistence during his study of psittacosis, an infectious disease of Australian parrots. The problem that he encountered during his research on this subject was the fact that many wild parrots, despite their healthy-looking appearance, were heavily infected with the psittacosis pathogen. These parrots manifested symptoms only in certain environments, such as cages. Why, then, did the parrots show no symptoms in their natural habitats? According to Burnet, they could remain healthy in so far as they remained in the places where they and the pathogen evolved together for a long time. Parrots and the psittacosis pathogen became adapted to each other in their wild environment and could thus maintain a kind of "equilibrium." But the situation could differ in artificial surroundings. In particular, in cages, which were "crowded, filthy, and without exercise or sunlight," the parrots could suffer from "a flare-up of any latent infection" [34]. The changed environmental condition, which altered the state of the host body, started the severe symptoms of psittacosis infection.

The existence of "intermediate hosts" suggested the same issue. While Burnet already knew of the intermediate hosts of malaria or yellow fever, his own study of Q-fever and his reading of the papers on Rocky Mountain spotted fever led him to raise a serious question—which was asked by few scholars—about the etiology and epidemiology of ticks, lice, or rats [35]. Why didn't these intermediate hosts suffer from infectious disease even though they held viruses, bacteria, and rickettsiae pathogenic to humans? Burnet wrote that the intermediate hosts did not become sick by contacting the microbes, because these two groups of organisms had become adapted to each other during their long coevolution [33, 36]. Since promoting their mutual survival and proliferation was beneficial to both groups, the force of evolution made the one's body unharmed by its contact with the other's. But the situation could change with humans' intrusion into this harmonized world. Since humans had not been adapted to this peaceful relationship, they could become severely ill after being infected with the microbes in the wild, even though the lice, the ticks, or the rat, which had carried them for a long time, would hardly become sick. With this conclusion, he further departed from the traditional germ theory of disease established in the late nineteenth century.

Burnet's research on the host-parasite interaction and his new ideas on disease were more clearly stated in his famous monograph, *Biological Aspects of Infectious Disease* (1940) [34]. As philosopher and historian of science Alfred I. Tauber has pointed out, Burnet, in writing this book, was influenced by H. G. Wells, Julian Huxley, and G. P. Wells' *The Science of Life* (1929) [7, 37]. Indeed, Wells, Huxley, and Wells' semi-popular book discussed many ecological subjects—such as succession, symbiosis, and food chain—along with healthy carrier problems and other medical issues which partially guided Burnet's idea on natural balance between the host and the parasite in the wild. But his own virological and bacteriological research was at least as important as *The Science of Life* in formulating his ecological ideas suggested in *Biological Aspects of Infectious Disease*. As historians J. Andrew Mendelsohn and Stephen Kunitz have shown, ecological perspectives in medical science, which viewed infectious disease as a disturbance of natural balance between the host and the parasite, originated during the early twentieth century within medical science itself rather than through the influence of ecologists upon medical experts [38-40]. As a person trained in medical research, his unique view of infectious disease explained in his book also reflected his own medical investigation, especially that concerning the host-parasite relationship.

Burnet proposed his first notion of "self" and "tolerance" in *Biological Aspects of Infectious Disease*. For Burnet, every living organism had to keep the boundary of its "self," because it played the role of both predator and prey in its food chains. Since each organism as a predator had to eat and digest others to survive, it had to maintain its distinction from the preys that should be consumed as food. Protozoa's destruction of bacteria in their vacuoles was a typical example, since the former digested only the latter without harming their own bodily component. Sometimes, however, the prey could evade the digestive system of the predator and attack it. If this were to happen, the "prey" could no longer be called a prey but should be considered a pathogen that would cause infectious disease in the host body. But Burnet thought that such an incident did not frequently happen in a large scale in a balanced natural state. Borrowing ecologists' term, Burnet argued that the host-pathogen relationship tended to develop into peaceful coexistence, which might be called the "climax" state. The climax was reached during evolution, because it was beneficial to every organism to promote the survival and steady proliferation of life including its own. In this state, "tolerance" between the host and the pathogen could be sustained until any extrinsic factor disturbed the balance.

In retrospect, Burnet was not alone in proposing the notion of "self" in immunity and disease, although his idea was different from that of other researchers. As historians and philosophers Alfred Tauber, Scott Podolsky, Ilana Löwy, and Kenton Kroker have argued, several medical and biological scientists already proposed diverse versions of the notion of "identity," "individuality," "integrity," or "self" during the early twentieth century [7, 8, 41, 42]. Transplantation biologist Leo Loeb argued that "individuality differentials" were determined by nuclear genes. The French physiologist and Nobel laureate Charles Richet also discussed individuality in terms of anaphylactic response against pathogens, and the Russian zoologist Elie Metchnikoff had a notion of organismic integrity which was defined during developmental process. As will be discussed in the next section, Medawar, too, gave a talk about individuality or "self-specificity" at Oxford University in 1946. While it is not clearly known how Burnet's idea of "self" in 1940 was related to these terms, we may assume as a broad reader of medical literature he was influenced by them in some degree. But Burnet differed from these scholars in conceiving the notion of self in an ecological sense, which was derived from his own medical investigation of the relationship between the host and the pathogen.

In *Biological Aspects of Infectious Disease*, Burnet discussed many issues regarding the host-pathogen interaction, which included the importance of the host body in the causation of disease. He wrote, "It will be obvious that the fatal result of any infection will depend both on the micro-organism and the host, and we can also feel certain that, except for certain abnormally fatal epidemics, the state of the host is of far greater importance in determining the outcome than is the virulence of the micro-organism." For instance, he explained the occurrence of puerperal fever as a result of the disturbed condition of the postpartum uterus rather than the invasion of *Streptococcus* which had traditionally been considered the causal agent. He also accounted for meningitis as resulting from the movement of *meningococcus* and other related bacteria from the throat to the brain. While these bacteria were mostly harmless in their natural habitat, the throat, they could bring about severe illness if they were to be accidentally placed in the brain. Another important phenomenon with related mechanism and implication was anaphylaxis. He stated that it occurred when the antibodies against a specific antigen—which came to be fixed in various parts of the body after the first infection—provoked an overly strong immune response after the second or later invasion of the antigen. According to him, this response could be a more important cause of the symptoms of many infectious diseases than pathogenic organisms themselves. For instance, he thought, the tubercle bacillus was only a partial cause of tuberculosis, since 80% of infected people did not develop any symptoms of the disease during their life. Hence, there must be other factors which determined the occurrence of tuberculosis for the unfortunate 20%. He supposed that anaphylaxis in the host body, along with its genetic constitution, should be an actual factor that caused the pathological symptoms of tuberculosis and even death. Many patients contracted tuberculosis, not because the tubercle bacillus invaded their body, but because they responded to it too vigorously.

As historian Ohad Parnes has shown, Burnet was not the only scientists in advocating this view [43]. After the early twentieth century, an increasingly large number of medical researchers were focusing on the role of the host body in the occurrence of infectious disease, and Burnet's idea reflected this new trend in medicine. These researchers were asking a question that had seldom been raised by doctors in earlier generations. Why did the parasites harm the host, if they could not get any benefit by doing so? It was certain that the germ did not have any *intention* to make the host sick. Therefore, the cause of disease had to be found elsewhere, especially in the interrelationship between the germ and the host rather than the mere existence of the germ within the host's body. This new awareness about the host body's role and its relation to the germ in disease causation gradually made the etiology of infection complex [38].

Burnet's immunological theory pertained to this concern about the host body. Like his London advisors Ledingham and Arkwright, Burnet thought that varying consequences of viral and bacterial infection were related to the state of the immune system of the host body. It was thus necessary to study the system more thoroughly, especially with regard to the production of antibodies and the mechanisms of establishing "self" and inducing "tolerance." Yet the most intensively discussed subjects in immunology were different at that time. As historian Arthur Silverstein and others have pointed out, immunology during the early and mid-twentieth century was dominated by "chemical immunologists" such as Felix Haurowitz and S. Mudd, who were more interested in molecular aspects of antigen-antibody reaction than complex biological dimensions of immunity concerning the whole body [8, 10, 12]. Burnet challenged this chemical orientation in immunology, and tried to conceive a new theory based on his biological thinking.

Burnet's second book, *The Production of Antibodies* (1941), provided an early version of this theory [44]. He criticized chemical immunologists' "template theory" which claimed that antibodies were formed by being pressed against an antigen that functioned as a physical "template." For Burnet, there were at least two problems in this theory. First, the template theory failed to explain the clinical observation that antibodies could be made even after the antigen was completely eliminated within the body. Second, the theory could not account for the fact that the immune reaction against an antigen became stronger when it entered the host body again. Hence, borrowing the recent biochemical research by René Dubos, Oswald Avery, Max Bergmann, and Carl Niemann, Burnet proposed a new theoretical idea. Initially, he postulated that reticulo-endothelial cells had a special enzyme that could synthesize itself and adapt its structure to the shapes of foreign antigens that it had digested in the cells. According to him, the adapted structure of this enzyme was retained while it reproduced itself and was "inherited" by two daughter cells as the original cell containing it divided. At the same time, the reticulo-endothelial cells released the enzyme's "partial replica," which would become the antibody in bloodstream. Thus, as long as the cells were alive, they could continue to produce the antibody against a specific antigen even if the antigen was no longer present in the body. The antibody-producing adaptive enzyme in the cells had already learned the antigen's structure. Furthermore, the repeated invasion of the antigen could produce antibodies with an enhanced reactivity, as the self-synthesizing adaptive enzyme became more closely adapted to the structure of the antigen.

In fact, this theory had many problems, if compared with his later theory proposed in the second edition of *The Production of Antibodies* (1949). Burnet claimed that his theory was better than the chemical theories, because it took into account the clinical aspects and the cellular mechanisms of immunity formation. But the limitations of his early theory were obvious to many readers, especially to those who read *Biological Aspects of Infectious Disease* as well. The most significant problem was that his theory did not account for how the immunological "self" of an organism was distinguished from that of other living creatures. How could the special enzyme within reticulo-endothelial cells could selectively destroy an antigen and become adapted to its shape, while leaving other molecules and cells within the body untouched? Another problem was that his theory did not mention anything about the peaceful relationship between the host and the parasite emphasized in *Biological Aspects of Infectious Disease*. How and why did the special enzyme within reticulo-endothelial cells fail to respond to certain antigens even though they were not originally a part of the host body? Probably, Burnet thought that the evolutionary adaptation of two or more organisms, which he tried to detail in *Biological Aspects of Infectious Disease*, was too complex to be described at the level of the antigen-antibody reaction.

But the first edition of *Production of Antibodies* did deal with a subject mentioned in *Biological Aspects of Infectious Disease*, namely, the problem of "tolerance." He cited James Murphy of the Rockefeller Institute, who observed that chick embryos did not respond to transplanted tumor tissues [45]. In fact, this discovery was highly meaningful at that time, because no one before Murphy had succeeded in transplanting extrinsic tissues to an organism without provoking adverse responses in the recipient except for a few special cases involving the cornea and other organs. Yet Murphy's chickens did reject the tumor tissue after they grew up, just as most adult human bodies failed to accept tissues from a different person. Burnet also noted that since James Murphy's work, several researchers proved that immature animals could receive outside transplants and infectious agents without violent resistance, although they rejected these extraneous entities after they became adults. To Burnet, these were examples of "tolerance" of an immature animal toward extrinsic agents due to its lack of fully developed immune system.

Although the meaning of "tolerance" in these statements was different from that in *Biological Aspects of Infectious Disease*, Burnet's emphasis on the host body could still be seen. Whereas Burnet explained "tolerance" in 1940 as a consequence of evolutionary adaptation over a long time span, the term designated in 1941 a temporary phenomenon due to the immaturity of the immune system of the host body. It is hard to explain why Burnet used the term differently in his two books. Perhaps he did not yet intend to use "tolerance" as a technical term in immunology with a cldar definition. Nevertheless, his 1941 book on antibody formation contained a core notion which was consistent with his deep interest in the host body's role in disease causation. Indeed, according to Burnet, young animals mentioned in his book did not respond to an extrinsic agent, because they were too young and immature. This revealed that the *age* of the host organism was a critical factor in determining the occurrence of disease.

Biological Aspects of Infectious Disease and his other publications contained extensive discussions of the "age-incidence of infectious disease." Burnet wrote that age, together with race, sex, nutritional state, and other factors, played a critical role in determining whether an infected host would develop pathological symptoms or not. His earliest interest in the factor of age can be found his investigation of the Bundaberg tragedy, which revealed that the survivors tended to be older than those who died. This implied that older children had a more mature immune system that protected them from being overwhelmed by a strain of *Staphylococcus* injected into their body. It is also significant that he had been using chick embryos to culture various viruses from the 1930s. These embryos, probably because they were extremely young, did not show any immune response to the viruses which were not their inherent parts. Burnet found interesting examples of the involvement of age from other researchers' publications as well. From the epidemiological data, he learned that influenza, yellow fever, and tuberculosis affected children more severely than young adults. Texas cattle fever, which was studied by the renowned American microbiologist Theobald Smith, showed a similar epidemiological pattern [46]. Adult cattle infected by the pathogenic protozoa tended to suffer more severe pathological symptoms than young calves.

Burnet's poliovirus research and his reading of other medical literature also led him to ponder how the age of the host body pertained to the evolutionary variation of the virus in relation to the changes of environment [47]. Burnet wrote that before the early twentieth century polio had been a mild disease affecting only the pharyngeal region of infants. During these past years, the poliovirus was not very virulent, since a mutually beneficial relationship between the virus and the human had been established. For the virus, the human body offered a good residential place and the nutrition for its survival and further proliferation. For humans, the poliovirus provided the immunity to more virulent strains without leading to severe pathological conditions. But after the initiation of modern public health movements and improved hygiene in the early twentieth century, this harmonious coexistence broke down. Since babies' health began to be more carefully managed by their parents in a cleaner environment, they were less likely to be infected by the poliovirus than those in earlier times. Consequently, a large group of children and young adults appeared with no experience of contacting the poliovirus in their younger age. In this state, the virus could undergo rapid proliferation and evolution if it had a chance to enter this group which had no immunity to polio. According to Burnet, this caused a huge disaster, because a mutant strain of the virus, which appeared through numerous passages into susceptible individuals, came to affect the brain and the spinal cord of the children and young adults who would subsequently undergo paralysis or death. This virulent form of the poliovirus and its changed "age-incidence" was a byproduct of altering the natural balance between the virus and the human through artificial measure in the name of public health and hygiene.

What, then, can be generalized from these diverse cases concerning the role of age of the host organism in the occurrence of infectious diseases? It was not easy to make a general statement on the subject, because the mode by which the age of the host functioned in disease causation was distinct in each case. In particular, the case of polio was different from other instances of infectious diseases, since its age-incidence was changed not by the alteration of the host body's state during growth but by the evolutionary variation of the virus.

Nevertheless, Burnet thought that it was possible to describe a general tendency that could be observed in many kinds of infectious disease. According to him, younger hosts tended to have a higher chance of avoiding fatal consequences of infection than older individuals. While it was often thought that "children are more prone to the common infections than adults because they are weaker," the epidemiological data of yellow fever, tuberculosis, human psittacosis, and influenza indicated that children's mortality rate was lower than that of young adults [34]. Even diseases affecting cattle revealed the same pattern as Smith showed through his Texas cattle fever study. Of course, there was no simple linear relationship between the host's age and mortality rate. As Burnet knew well, it was found that older children had a better chance of survival in the Bundaberg tragedy. Moreover, it was generally known that among younger groups of hosts infants had a higher mortality in infectious disease than children. Nevertheless, the general tendency which was favorable toward younger people was obvious. Whereas infants showed a higher rate of death than children, they had a lower mortality than young adults. The survival of older children in the Bundaberg tragedy must reflect a minor variation within the younger hosts.

Burnet offered an immunological and evolutionary explanation on this age-incidence of infectious disease. The reason why adults had a higher mortality could be found in their body's overly strong response, which may include anaphylaxis against pathogenic microbes. Although this response was formed during evolution in order to help adult humans survive after injuries and local traumas during their hunting activity, it came to affect their own body adversely in an infection with certain viruses or bacteria, especially those that the adults had not encountered in their younger age. In contrast, children, who did not yet have this excessively potent response toward microbes, could adequately deal with extrinsic agents with their moderately developed immune system. Since their immune response was neither too strong nor too weak, they tended to have a better chance of survival than other age groups. The case of infants stood between that of adults and children. While their immune system was often too weak to respond to all the microbes appropriately, it was not overly strong and could not thus overwhelm their own body.

But what was the case of even younger hosts, such as the fetus or the embryo? As I have written, Burnet used chick embryos as a culture medium of his viruses, and was well aware of James Murphy and others' research on embryonic animals' "immature" immune response to extrinsic cells and microbes. While scientific research on this subject was not yet extensive, Burnet thought that it was very important for a further elucidation of the role of the host body in the occurrence of infectious diseases.

Burnet's deep interest in this problem led him to accept cytoplasmic inheritance theories, which seemed to provide a satisfactory theoretical framework for conceptualizing what is happening in a developing embryonic body [48-49]. As historian Jan Sapp has described, cytoplasmic inheritance was championed by a number of renowned biologists during the 1940s, including Tracy Sonneborn, C. D. Darlington, Sol Spiegelman, and Carl and Gertrude Lindegren [50]. As we will see in the next section, Peter Medawar also supported cytomplasmic inheritance through his tissue transplantation experiments. Criticizing geneticists' claim that the nucleus was the only organelle with the genetic material, these researchers argued that hereditary entities could also be found within the cytoplasm whose function was at least partially independent of the genes in the nucleus. According to the supporters of cytoplasmic inheritance, the hereditary materials in the cytoplasm were the agents responsible for cell differentiation during embryogenesis. Although regular geneticists argued that nuclear genes guided the differentiation of cell types and developmental process, this argument was not very persuasive to many biologists at that time. Since almost every somatic cell of a multicellular organism had the same set of nuclear genes, it should be the cytoplasm rather than the nucleus that made the difference among distinct cellular types. It was also important that this difference was not pre-established before conception but was formed gradually during developmental phases. Of course, the champions of cytoplasmic inheritance did not argue that cell differentiation was completely independent of the influence of nuclear genes. Rather, they argued that embryogenesis and cell differentiation were complex phenomena involving the constant interactions among cytoplasmic hereditary entities, nuclear genes, and environmental factors within the intercellular space. More specifically, they thought, cytoplasmic hereditary entities, which must have been initially made by nuclear genes, underwent gradual transformations during development by contacting other cells and changing intercellular environments. These transformed cytoplasmic factors would be inherited by two daughter cells that would undergo further proliferation under the influence of their surroundings and other cells. Through this process during growth, the type of each cell was gradually determined.

To Burnet, cytoplasmic inheritance theories were highly useful, because they enabled him to extend his previous hypothesis of antibody formation proposed in 1941. The reticulo-endothelial enzymes in 1941, which could digest and become adapted to foreign antigens, could now be placed in the cytoplasm of immune cells and be regarded as one of their hereditary entities. But what was important was not just the enzyme's location within the cell. Cytoplasmic inheritance theories furnished the enzyme with a *temporal dimension* that could be employed in explaining the formation of immunological "self" [12]. As I have written, Burnet hoped to understand varying behaviors of the host according to its age. Especially, he became interested in the immune response of the youngest host to viruses and bacteria due to Murphy's and others' experiments and his use of the chick embryo as a viral culture medium. With this interest in mind, he provisionally accepted cytoplasmic inheritance theories for a further conceptualization of antibody formation of developing animals. The changes of the adaptive enzymes in the reticulo-endothelial cells could now be explained in terms of growing organisms' dynamic process of adapting their cytoplasmic components to changing inner environments. This theoretical model would be used to explain very young animals' curious immunological and etiological behavior.

With regard to this behavior, some interesting observational cases began to appear in scientific and medical literature of the 1930s and 1940s. In his

1945 paper, Ray Owen at the University of Wisconsin wrote that he conducted an extensive blood testing of cows that had twin brother or sister coming from a distinct egg [51]. Knowing that the "freemartin," the infertile young female cow, was made through vascular anastomosis between dizygotic twin calves during embryogenesis and fetal phase, he argued that the shared blood circulation during these periods also caused many dizygotic twin calves' identical blood types observed by him. This was an interesting finding in terms of immunology, because it was known that two genetically distinct cows could hardly have the same blood type due to the large number of different kinds of blood antigens in cattle. Based on this fact and other evidence, Owen construed that the dizygotic twins' identical types of blood cells were the descendents of the embryonic and fetal cells that had been exchanged between the two fetuses in a uterus. During their early life, the cattle learned not to respond to the blood cells of distinct genetic constitution coming from their dizygotic twin brother or sister. Another important observational case relevant to Burnet's theoretical commitment was published by Erich Traub at the Rockefeller Institute for Medical Research. In a series of papers published in the 1930s, Traub described that his mice infected with the choriomeningitis virus in their embryonic stages could not provoke immune response against the virus even after their developmental phase had ended [52-54]. Like Owen's research, Traub showed an example of young organisms' nonresponse to extrinsic agent which could be extended to adult phases.

Burnet cited these two studies in the second edition of *Production of Antibodies* (1949) with the cooperation of his colleague Frank Fenner [1]. Burnet and Fenner wrote that Owen's and Traub's findings were key examples of the theory of "self" and "tolerance," because both implied that any extrinsic entity that had entered the host body during its embryonic and fetal stage could be regarded as its "self" and thus be permanently "tolerated." Although Burnet and Fenner suggested further experimental research regarding the theory of "self," Owen's and Traub's work implied that Burnet's idea was already supported by strong empirical evidence.

As Alfred Tauber and Scott Podolsky have pointed out, however, the actual role of Owen's and Traub's studies in Burnet's conception of his theory should not be exaggerated [7]. Although several scientists, such as Ian R. Mckay, Gustav Nossal, and Alberto Martini, have argued that Burnet arrived at his mature theory of "self" and "tolerance" in 1949 directly through these observations by Owen and Traub, they did not take into account the broader context of Burnet's research [3-5]. First, they did not explain why Burnet became interested in Owen's and Traub's papers in the first place. Among a large number of published papers Burnet read, why were Owen's and Traub's articles so important to him? This question becomes more curious, if we see the difference between Owen's and Traub's investigations in their historical context. During the 1930s and 1940s, what Traub found was considered a classical case of the balanced coexistence between the host and the parasite which Burnet extensively discussed in *Biological Aspects of Infectious Disease*, while Owen's observation was a curious phenomenon in which immunological barrier was completely ignored. In fact, the nature of extraneous entity was different in the two instances: In Traub's work, it was a virus that could infect a mammalian host, whereas Owen dealt with red blood cells without such a capacity. Hence, while it could be taken for granted that red blood cells would not harm the calves by themselves, it could still be asked why the choriomeningitis virus did not attack the mice. Although the host's response was similar in the two cases, the extrinsic agent's nature and expected behavior was totally different. As we will see, Medawar did not cite Traub in his famous paper of 1953, probably because he felt that Traub's study was not relevant to his tissue transplantation experiment. In contrast, Burnet viewed the two phenomena in a single theoretical standpoint.

What, then, made Burnet treat these two seeming distinct topics in a single theory? I think that it was his medical training and subsequent study in microbiology and epidemiology. Burnet did not think that a microbial infection always led to a disease. Most microbes, including both bacteria and viruses, were harmless in their natural habitats. For this reason, an infection of mice with the choriomeningitis virus was not very different from the intrusion of genetically distinct blood cells into fetal calves. Since Burnet did not ask why the virus did not harm or kill the mice in Traub's study, the crucial difference between Traub's and Owen's works, which was obvious to some later or contemporary readers, became insignificant to him.

For Burnet, the two studies were also similar in terms of the common role *age* played in the host body's response. In both Traub's and Owen's observations, the host body came to contact extrinsic agents in fetal and embryonic stages, in which Burnet had been deeply interested throughout his career. As I have written, he had been concerned about what he called the "age-incidence of infectious disease" in *Biological Aspects of Infectious Disease*. In this book, he pondered how the response of a host body to pathogens could differ according to its age. Likewise, the second edition of *Production of Antibodies* (1949) included a chapter on "Immunological Behavior of Young Animals," which discussed various issues related to the age-incidence of the host body's behavior concerning extrinsic agents. In this chapter, he wrote that "there is abundant clinical evidence that certain human infections (e.g. typhus) have a much higher mortality in old persons than in children or young adults" [1]. It also seemed quite important that "all who have investigated the skin reactions of children to bacterial toxins have noted the absence of reaction in very young infants." Experimental studies of embryos and fetuses were important as well. Burnet discussed Murphy's and later researchers' observations of the nonresponse of embryonic hosts, and mentioned his own work on chick embryos infected with influenza virus. An important new example in this list of peculiar responses of young hosts was provided by Owen. He wrote that "the important implication of this work is that cells 'foreign' to the host may be tolerated indefinitely provided they are implanted early in embryonic life."

Burnet used cytoplasmic inheritance theories in theorizing the mechanism of this process. He first postulated that every cell in an embryo had a "self-marker" which was genetically determined. Yet this marker could function only when it was recognized by self-replicating adaptive enzymes, which were a kind of cytoplasmic hereditary material within phagocytes. During embryogenesis, as phagocytes wandered over the body and engulfed various cells and molecules, the adaptive enzymes within them could destroy the self-marker on each cell and become adapted to its shape. Since the enzymes with this adapted form would be inherited by daughter phagocytes while replicating themselves within the cytoplasm, at the end of embryogenesis, all kinds of the self-marker in the body would have been memorized by the enzymes through their altered structure. In this state, an extrinsic molecule or cell entering the developed body could not "fit" with the structure of the self-replicating adaptive enzymes. Hence, the enzymes would recognize the molecule or cell as "foreign" and be converted to the "primary units" whose "partial replica" would be released as antibodies in bloodstream. But even this foreign entity could be recognized as a part of the "self" if it had been implanted within the body during its embryonic and fetal phase. Self-replicating adaptive enzymes within phagocytes would then be adapted to the shape of the foreign entity and would recognize it thereafter as a part of the "self." Through this mechanism, Burnet argued, "the process by which self-pattern becomes recognizable takes place during the embryonic or immediately post-embryonic stages." Even a foreign entity with no genetic relation to the host body could then be permanently "tolerated" after the end of its embryo and fetal stages.

This hypothetical mechanism reflected his view of life which had been constantly developing after he finishing his Ph.D. dissertation 1928. While the concept of "self" changed from an ecological notion in 1940 to an immunological one in 1949 based on the functions of the adaptive enzymes and the self-markers, the new theory still contained Burnet's core philosophy. The interior of an animal's body was a harmonized world in which the self-replicating adaptive enzymes and the self-markers became gradually adapted to each other during embryogenesis. This was highly similar to the climax state in the wild consisted of predators and preys that were adapted to each other, as he described in *Biological Aspects of Infectious Disease* in 1940. The events occurring after a foreign entity entered these harmonized worlds were also very similar. In the case of wild nature, the intrusion of foreign organisms, such as humans, could disrupt its natural balance and induce infectious diseases. In the case of an animal body, a foreign molecule or cell could provoke an immune response, because it did not fit with the shape of the self-replicating enzymes that were perfectly adapted to the structure of the host body's self-markers. In these two worlds, even the mechanism of establishing tolerance was alike, since in both cases a certain time span and the gradual adaptation of an outside agent were required. In the wild nature, the balance that had been disturbed by an outside agent could be restored and the climax state could be reestablished, as the agent gradually began to be regarded as a part of the system. Within an animal body, an extrinsic agent that entered the host body during embryogenesis and fetal development could be indefinitely considered a part of the "self" by changing the shape of the self-replicating adaptive enzyme over time.

Burnet hoped that his theory could be experimentally demonstrated. Although it was already being supported by Owen's and Traub's findings, an experimental inoculation of a foreign antigen into an embryo or fetus would provide stronger proof of his idea. He wrote,

> The self-marker concept seems to provide a number of suggestions for experimental work to substantiate or refute it. A virtually direct proof of its correctness could be obtained if experimental techniques could be developed to produce with a wider range of antigens introduced into embryos the persisting tolerance of foreign cells found by Owen in his studies on multiple births in cattle [1].

In 1950, Burnet and his Australian colleagues tried to demonstrate his theory using the chick embryo [55]. In designing their experiments, Burnet and his team thought that three kinds of extrinsic entities injected into a chick embryo—influenza virus A, bacterial virus C16, and human red blood cells—would not only be indefinitely tolerated but also make the chicken receive the same entity after its growth without generating antibody response.

Unfortunately, this experiment did not show what he wanted to see. All the animals that had been inoculated with the viruses and red blood cells invariably produced violent antibody reactions after being challenged by the same agents in the sixth week after hatching.

After this failure in experimental demonstration, Burnet's 1949 theory itself had to be abandoned, too. In 1957, two years after the Danish scientist Niels K. Jerne proposed his "natural selection theory of antibody formation" [56], Burnet suggested the "clonal selection theory" that completely replaced his 1949 hypothesis [57]. The new theory postulated a totally different mechanism of constructing "self" and inducing "tolerance" based on the Darwinian principle applied to the cells in the immune system. Since this theory has been shown to have strong experimental supports, it has emerged as a paradigmatic theory in immunology which can explain the formation of antibodies, the construction of immunological self, and the production of tolerance.

But the failure of his 1949 theory does not mean that it was meaningless within the history of science. Although the making of "self" and "tolerance" is explained differently by the clonal selection theory, his 1949 argument that immunological self is defined during early developmental period has still been valid. Moreover, even before the proposal of the clonal selection theory, Peter Medawar in England published an influential paper in 1953 which gave a strong support to Burnet's 1949 theory. Yet it is not true that Medawar conducted his experiments only as a means to prove Burnet's idea. The next section will show that Medawar pursued his immunological research through a distinct methodology and perspective that had originated from his unique academic training and professional career.

Chapter 3

GROWTH, AGING, AND TISSUE TRANSPLANTATION IN PETER BRIAN MEDAWAR'S RESEARCH

Peter Medawar was born in Rio de Janeiro, Brazil in 1915 and was educated in Magdalen College at the University of Oxford from 1932 to 1936. There he finished his undergraduate education with a "First" in zoology and worked as a demonstrator and research fellow before being appointed Mason Professor of Zoology at the University of Birmingham in 1947.

During his early career and education, Medawar was broadly interested in theoretical and mathematical aspects of the biological sciences. Through his theoretical study, Medawar became deeply concerned about the living organisms' changes over time—development, aging, and evolution—and their interrelations. A major influence on this growing academic interest was the British biologist D'Arcy W. Thompson (1860-1948)'s *On Growth and Form* (1917) [58]. Thompson's book taught him that various living organisms' growth and the geometric relationship of their changing morphology could be mathematically described and studied. Medawar also incorporated the tools of biostatistics and the new evolutionary theories after the Modern Synthesis through Ronald A. Fisher, Julian Huxley, J. B. S. Haldane, Alfred J. Lotka, and other scientists. He came to learn how evolution could be understood through natural selection and be explained using statistical analyses. As we will see, his use of these scientists' mathematical techniques and theoretical ideas substantially contributed to the construction of his evolutionary theory of aging.

Medawar absorbed his colleagues' thoughts and practices through his education and social networks. He regularly corresponded with Thompson, who gave his comments on Medawar's papers to help him revise them for publication. Deeply appreciating this help and the insights he gained from Thompson's book, Medawar wrote a chapter in *Essays on Growth and Form Presented to D'Arcy Wentworth Thompson* (1945), edited by Wilfred E. Le Gros Clark and Medawar himself [59]. Medawar also knew Fisher in person and asked him to furnish his mice for the tissue transplantation research. Fisher gladly offered his mice, and like Thompson, helped Medawar by reading and commenting on Medawar's papers, one of which was transmitted to *The Proceedings of the Royal Society* through Fisher's recommendation [60]. Medawar also became aware of other contributors to the Modern Synthesis through his Oxford alumni-faculty network. Indeed, as Jack Morrell has shown, many prominent evolutionary scientists taught and studied at the University of Oxford during the early and mid-twentieth century, including Huxley, Haldane, Edward Poulton, E. S. Goodrich, and E. B. Ford [61]. An article titled "Oxford Zoology" written by Medawar in 1944 shows that he deeply respected these biologists and their research, and regarded himself as a member of this actively growing scientific community [62].

Medawar's first published paper based on his early research at Howard Florey's physiology lab shows how Medawar began to use mathematical and theoretical approaches he learned from these scholars to analyze a biological phenomenon, namely, "ageing" of tissues explanted from embryonic animals. Although his first paper, which was basically his D. Phil. degree thesis, did not contain any mathematical formulas, he nevertheless tried to account for his experimental results in quantitative terms. In this paper, he summarized his study of the biological properties of a factor in malt extracts that had been known to inhibit the proliferation of cells. He observed that the susceptibility of explanted tissue to the inhibitory effects of the factor increased with the tissue's age. This observation led him to think that the "growth energy" of tissues could be represented as the capacity to grow under the influence of the inhibitory factor [63]. Younger tissues with more growth energy tended to grow at a higher rate than older tissues in the presence of the same amount of the inhibitory factor.

In his second article published in 1940, he studied this phenomenon further with carefully designed experiments and mathematical analyses. He wrote that the growth energy of tissues increased in proportion to the concentration of the inhibitory factor that was *"just sufficiently high* to inhibit all [outgrowths] from a series of explants of differing embryonic ages" [64].

He then actually measured these concentrations using the explanted embryonic chicken heart aged from 6 to 18 days, and from this observational data, determined the growth energy and its mathematical relation to the heart's age.

But what was more important in this 1940 paper was the "specific growth rate," together with the relationship between the mass of the tissue and its age. Medawar thought that the specific growth rate, which was defined as the rate of change of mass divided by the current mass, was in direct proportion to the growth energy. From this idea and an equation based on it, he deduced the relationship between the mass of the embryonic chicken heart tissue and its age: $W = W_i\, e^{-ae^{-kt}}$. This meant that "the heart of the chicken grows *at a rate of continuous compound interest which itself declines by continuous compound interest*" [64]. That is, while the growth of the tissue occurred exponentially through the duplication of existing cells, the rate of this duplication decreased exponentially over time. For Medawar, this was a characteristic of *senescence*, which proceeded even during embryo development.

In a broader perspective, Medawar's conclusion challenged the traditional notion of aging process and gave support to the American embryologist Charles S. Minot's paradoxical statement. While it had been thought that humans went through the periods of "growing up" and "growing old," Medawar's research on the aging of embryonic tissues implied that no such distinction was meaningful in scientific understanding of senescence. Aging proceeded even in the earliest stages of life. In fact, a similar idea had already been proposed by Minot in 1908. Based on his observation of the chicken's growth rates, he had argued that the rate of the decline of growth rate was highest in the early phase of an organism's life and gradually slowed down in its later course [65]. Since Minot regarded the decline of growth as a symptom of aging, his observation was led to his paradoxical conclusion that aging not only occurred during early life, but also proceeded then at the highest speed. In 1941, Medawar cited this idea of Minot and argued that his tissue culture experiment supported it. The phenomenon of senescence was no longer limited to the later portions of life, because growth always accompanied senile changes. Moreover, the fact that the "specific acceleration of growth $d/dt\,(dw/Wdt)$, while always negative, rises progressively to zero during the course of life" vindicated Minot's claim that "organisms age fastest when they are young" [66]. This topic would be referred again in his later research on aging and immunological tolerance.

Another paper published in 1943, titled "The Shape of the Human Being as a Function of Time," shows how Medawar tried to describe this age change—whether it meant growth or senescence—in mathematical terms [60]. While his previous works concerned only the cell's growth and aging, this article dealt with those of the whole human being, particularly the change of the relative proportion of its parts with aging. Citing the books of Thompson and Huxley whose methodology Medawar adopted in the paper, he suggested a mathematical way to describe the growth of a man in accordance with his age. Using a series of pictures showing his growth process only as the changing bodily proportion without altering the actual height, he traced the distance of four portions of the body (the fork, navel, nipples, and chin) from the base-line in mathematical terms using a function of time. According to his equation, if two variables—time and the initial distance of a body part from the base-line—were to be known, it was possible to predict the location of the part at that time. Medwar thought that by creating this equation he succeeded in describing each part's growth "as a single process of continuous deformation in time."

For Medawar, however, writing this kind of paper was not his major activity. In a letter to Fisher, Medawar wrote that he completed the above paper "in [his] spare time from medical research." According to Medawar's recollection, this medical research was initiated with the beginning of World War II through his study of the restoration of severed peripheral nerves. While pursuing this work, he also investigated other related issues, such as the effects and toxicity of sulfonamide drugs and the proper way of using fixatives for the treatment of burned skin [67, 68]. But the most important job for him at the time was the research on the "homograft problem" which he pursued with Thomas Gibson and Leonard Colebrook at the Burns Unit of the Glasgow Royal Infirmary [23]. Indeed, the use of skin homograft—a piece of the skin transplanted from a different person—for burned patients was attempted in many hospitals without much success. Although it was highly urgent to treat the patients severely burned during warfare, many of them did not have enough of their own skin that could be used to cover their damaged surface. Yet it was not possible to use the skin from a different person other than a monozygotic twin brother or sister, since it had already been known for a long time that such skin would be invariably rejected by the patient's body [69]. To investigate more basic causes of this problem, Medawar began his own research using rabbits and mice at Oxford with a small grant awarded by the Medical Research Council. He studied whether homograft rejection was caused by an immune reaction or by local cellular response. If the former was the case, it was necessary to determine whether the response occurred through an acquired immunity, which was normally used to protect the organism against microbial infection, or a "natural immunity," which was thought to be innate but magnified itself during blood transfusion [70]. He also investigated the genetic mechanism underlying the homograft rejection phenomenon through the inbred mice that he acquired from Fisher's laboratory.

Although Medawar's major scientific method in this war-related research was experimentation, mathematics was also important as an instrument of research design. For instance, he tried to determine the minimum number of antigens responsible for homograft rejection. Using the mathematical techniques of permutation and combination, he devised an experiment which aimed at testing if there were at least seven distinct antigens involved in the host body's response toward a homograft [71]. In this experiment, the number seven did not have much meaning. Although Medawar did not explain clearly, it was probably just a number that was chosen according to Medawar's practical constraint, especially the number of his available experimental animals. In fact, considering this constraint and based on his calculation using permutation and combination, he decided to use twenty-five rabbits to examine whether the number of antigen in homograft rejection was at least seven. He transplanted to each individual a piece of tissues from every other rabbit. According to Medawar's calculation, even a single case of successful transplantation and survival of the tissues could mean that the number of antigens was fewer than seven. Of course, it was also possible that two or more experimental rabbits shared the same genes for antigen production. In that case, further experimental studies would be necessary. Yet if all the tissues were rejected, then there must be more than seven antigens involved in homograft rejection. The result of his transplantation experiments indicated that this was indeed the case. Since every rabbit, except the two that died prematurely and the one excluded due to illness, rejected all the tissues that came from the other rabbits, he concluded that there were at least seven antigens responsible for rejecting homografts.

Whereas this conclusion was not followed by any further research on the number of antigens, it illustrates his way of approaching biological problems. Like the senior British scholars he respected such as Fisher, he analyzed the problems in a mathematical way and designed an experiment to answer a specific question regarding them. Admittedly, the above experiment did not produce any clues for a further experimental study. The finding that there were at least seven antigens involved in homograft rejection merely meant that the actual number of the antigens could be eight, nine, or a thousand. From our standpoint, it could be said that Medawar was approaching the problem in a wrong way. Yet it shows how he was treating the subjects in immunology. He problematized the subjects in terms of numbers and possibilities and conducted an experiment based on them. Although this kind of approach was frequently found among physical scientists, it was unusual for biologists, except for some British scholars Medawar knew well.

Medawar employed a similar methodology to infer the "tempo" of the breakdown of homografts from the changing number of surviving skin patches over time [72]. In this experiment, there were four experimental groups. The first was the group of rabbits that received the "low dosage" homograft from different rabbits, whereas the second was that which received the "high dosage." The third and fourth groups were those which experienced grafting of the same foreign tissues twice. Their difference was that while the third group got the second homograft at a body part different from the place where the first skin patch was transplanted the fourth had the second homograft attached to the very place where the first from the same donor was rejected. He arrived at two conclusions from this experiment. First, the cause of the homograft rejection was actively acquired immunity, since the second-set homograft was rejected more rapidly, as could be seen in the difference between the first and third groups. Second, the amount of grafted tissue had something to do with the pattern of rejection, as could be seen in the difference between the first and second groups in the same experiment. But what was the precise nature of this difference? To answer this question, Medawar used C. I. Bliss' statistical method of expressing "the percentages of graft mortality as areas of the normal curve of error in terms of the normal deviate" [72]. With this method, Medawar was able to calculate the "probit mortality," which, to put it simply, is the probability that a randomly chosen skin homograft would be dead by a specific date. By comparing the rate of the increase of the probit mortality of the first and second groups, Medawar concluded that "the *tempo* at which breakdown proceeds, once the process has started, is the same for both: the difference between them lies in the length of the latent period which must pass before the homograft reaction becomes effective." The amount of homograft skin tissue influenced only the brief period before the actual rejection process.

Medawar studied another phenomenon related to the living organism's changes over time—how the *age* of an organism influenced the regeneration of its peripheral nerves and the result of tissue transplantation—although he did not use any mathematics in investigating this issue. He and his colleagues studied the rate of regeneration of rabbits' severed peripheral nerves under varying conditions as a wartime research project, and found that young rabbits of one month old did not differ from adult rabbits in their rate of the advancement of the axon tip of a severed nerve cell, whereas the length of time required for the functional completion and the "scar delays," the time for a severed nerve fiber to retrogress before growing forward, were shorter in younger rabbits [73]. He also studied how the age of skin donors and recipients influenced the outcome of tissue transplantation. As we will see, this research was a crucial early work that formed a starting point of his later research on immune tolerance. However, this experiment itself did not seem to produce any new result that could interest Medawar. He found that young rabbits aged between 2½ and 4½ weeks old did not show any difference from adult rabbits in terms of homograft rejection. This result did not mean, however, that age was irrelevant in tissue transplantation. It simply implied that "the power of resistance to skin homografts is fully developed in rabbits ranging between 2½ and 4½ weeks in age" [71].

When, then, was the critical period in an organism's life, during which "the power of resistance to skin homografts" was formed? Like Burnet, Medawar suspected that embryogenesis was the period during which the capacity resist to foreign graft was formed. He was well aware of James Murphy's and others' early experiments which indicated that embryonic organism did not reject extrinsic agents. He thus felt that it was necessary to study the developmental period further to understand the nature of changes occurring in embryogenesis and the factors making the embryo accept agents of extrinsic origins without resistance. For Medawar, this research was important for another reason. The study of embryo development was a way to appreciate the repair process after injury, since the two processes—embryogenesis and tissue regeneration—resembled each other very closely. Since both entailed rapid cell proliferation in accordance with the shape of the whole body, the study of embryo growth was expected to produce results that could help his wartime projects on the regeneration of tissues [74].

As conceptual equipment for exploring embryo development, Medawar accepted cytoplasmic inheritance theories, just as Burnet did. Although some later scholars, along with Medawar himself in his old age, mentioned his employment of cytoplasmic inheritance theories as a serious "mistake" [14, 23], the theories during the 1940s played a certain role in his conceptualization of the connection among growth, pigment spread, and tissue transplantation. According to Medawar, the hereditary materials in the cytoplasm were probably the agent responsible for cell differentiation during embryogenesis, because "*all* the cells of the individual have the *same* complement of nuclear genes" [74]. It should thus be the cytoplasm rather than the nucleus that made the difference among distinct types of somatic cells. More specifically, cytoplasmic hereditary material underwent gradual transformation by contacting other cells and changing intercellular environments during embryonic and fetal phase. As this transformed cytoplasmic material replicated itself and was inherited by descendent cells, every cell containing this material in its cytoplasm would take a specific cell type after the end of developmental stage.

After leaving Oxford to become Mason Professor of Zoology at the University of Birmingham in 1947, Medawar and his colleague R. E. Billingham published their research on what they thought was a cytoplasmic inheritance material through their study of melanogenesis in guinea pig's skin. They argued that skin melanogenesis was caused by a self-replicating cytoplasmic hereditary entity and that such an entity also caused cell differentiation during embryogenesis [75]. Medawar and Billingham claimed that the migration of the self-replicating cytoplsmic entity to other cells and its subsequent proliferation offered the best explanation of the darkening of a white skin area into which a black guinea pig's skin was transplanted. In making this claim, Medawar did not forget to stress that cytoplasmic inheritance theories were championed by several renowned scholars such as Darlington, Sonneborn, and Spiegelman [76].

It is quite remarkable that Medawar's use of cytoplasmic inheritance was different from that of Burnet in at least two respects. First, Medawar conducted actual experiments on cytoplasmic inheritance which Burnet cited, whereas Burnet himself never designed or performed an experiment on hereditary entities within the cytoplasm. Second, Burnet's theoretical use of cytoplasmic inheritance at least partially contributed to his successful conceptualization of the formation of "self" during early life, while Medawar's study of cytoplasmic inheritance was not clearly connected to his theoretical concerns on immunological identity. These differences may raise a question. Do they support the widespread assumption that Burnet was a theoretician and Medawar was an experimentalist? In response to this question, I hope to stress the fact that Medawar's employment of cytoplasmic inheritance was connected to a specific research subject, skin pigmentation, which he could study using his expertise in tissue transplantation. Burnet, who did not have such a project, used cytoplasmic inheritance only as a theoretical tool for conceptualizing "self" and "tolerance." The distinct way of using cytoplasmic inheritance was pertained to the state of their research rather than their overall research orientation.

What, then, is Medawar's conceptual tool for his theorization of immunological identity? The remaining part of this monograph will show that Medawar, unlike Burnet, did not develop a specific theoretical model on the mechanism of the formation of "self." But Medawar, like Burnet, viewed the living organism as a dynamic entity that constantly changed itself through growth, aging, and evolution. This dynamic view of life contributed to both his evolutionary theory of aging and experiment on immunological tolerance.

Medawar first mentioned the issue of immunological "individuality," especially in terms of development and heredity during his 1946 lecture at the University of Oxford. It is not known whether Medawar was then aware of Burnet's early theories of "self" proposed in 1940. As I have written in the previous section, however, various versions of the idea of immunological identity had already been proposed by several scientists, and it is probable that Medawar read at least one of them. For him, the homograft rejection phenomenon and the problem of blood group incompatibility were the classical examples of the consequence of this individuality. According to him, "Individual differentiation or *self-specificity* develops," as could be seen from the fact that "the chick, before the eighteenth day of incubation, is almost indiscriminately hospitable" to extrinsic agents [77]. Yet the absence of homograft rejection among highly inbred animals meant that individuality had a genetic basis as well. Perhaps the making of immunological "self" was governed by both genes and developmental processes. He also thought that the antigen, after being made from nuclear genes, functioned as a kind of "self-reproducing *cytoplasmic genes*" whose structural incompatibility with the antibody provoked immune responses. During this lecture, however, Medawar did not suggest any further theoretical details about the basis of immunological self-specificity or the significance of "cytoplasmic genes."

Medawar argued that immunological individuality had an evolutionary as well as embryological dimension. He wrote that the rejection response toward a different individual's tissue was a byproduct of evolution, during which animals developed mechanisms of protecting themselves against invading microbes. While such mechanisms successfully increased the rate of survival of the individual and was thus selected during evolution, it came to frustrate surgeons' efforts to transplant homograft, even though the tissues of a distinct person did not "invade" the recipient's body as microbes did.

This evolutionary explanation of immunological individuality was different from that of Burnet. As I have written, Burnet did not take the "invasion" of microbes and the host's "protection" against them for granted. For him, the usual host-parasite relationship that developed during evolution was peaceful coexistence rather than hostile encounters involving invasion and protection. Based on his virological research and epidemiological inquiry, Burnet thought that a struggle between the host and the germ leading to infectious disease occurred only when the balance of nature was disturbed for some reasons. In contrast, Medawar, who did not study virology or epidemiology, held a more traditional view of infectious disease as an "invasion" of microbes.

However, Medawar was still similar to Burnet in terms of the broad interest in the organism's temporal dimensions, including development and evolution. Medawar wrote that "lower" animals in the evolutionary scale did not reject homograft just as "higher" organisms in their embryonic and fetal periods failed to resist extrinsic agents. According to him, "the rule that skin cannot be transplanted between individuals of the same species is known to be true only of higher vertebrates—from adult frogs and upwards.....though it sometimes seems to work in adult birds" [77]. This implied that "individuality" or "self-specificity," which was employed to distinguish one organism from another in infection and tissue transplantation, was something that developed over time during both embryogenesis and evolution. In a language reminiscent of the old biogenetic law of nineteenth century biology, he thus argued, "As self-specificity develops [during embryogenesis], so also it evolves."

This statement showed Medawar's view that all kinds of biological changes were interrelated. Just as aging did not need to be clearly distinguished from growth, the meaning of developmental process should not be completely dissociated from that of evolutionary changes. In 1951, he also published an article on the relationship between phylogeny (evolution) and ontogeny (embryogenesis). From his own observation, he argued that *Amphioxus* and the ascidian were very close in terms of phylogeny because they shared significant portions of the developmental process [78]. The shared growth process of the two species meant that they shared the evolutionary pathway as well.

But Medawar, who was sensitive to the new discoveries and conceptual innovations in contemporary biology, did not give any further support to the biogenetic law or recapitulation theory, which postulated that an organism's embryo and fetal development repeated its evolutionary history. Rather, he wholeheartedly accepted the new evolutionary biology after the Modern Evolutionary Synthesis completed during 1940s through the efforts of a number of scientists in Britain and America. As I have written, Medawar knew many distinguished British evolutionary biologists through his education at Oxford and his professional networks. From them, he absorbed the newly established notion that evolution is directionless, depending only upon random genetic mutation and natural selection within an environment where an organism happened to live.

Medawar's research memo shows that he adopted at least three new ideas proposed by the champions of the Modern Synthesis, many of whom were at Oxford. The first idea was Ford's, Huxley's, and Haldane's concept of the "time genes," which indicated that certain genes were activated only at or after a specific phase in an organism's life course [79-81]. The second idea, which partially included the first, was the American zoologist George G. Simpson's notion that "hereditary factors that reach their expression only after adults cease to breed have little bearing on natural selection" [82]. According to Simpson, such factors were subject to deleterious mutations that might bring about random variations when "only a fraction of the individuals survive in any case." The third was Fisher's "reproductive value," which was defined as the extent to which "persons of [a certain] age, on the average, contribute to the ancestry of future generations" per head [83].

Medawar created his own theoretical standpoint on aging using these three ideas as well as Minot's older argument, his tissue culture research, and a statement in Alfred Lotka's book. Based on Ford's, Huxley's, Haldane's, and Simpson's ideas, he concluded that the genes expressed in later phases of life could mutate without the influence of natural selection, making the changes occurring in these periods a kind of rudimentary alterations that had little to do with reproduction. But Medawar thought that there should be no given point of time when the "later phases of life" began [84]. As his tissue culture and Minot's study taught him, senescence occurred even in the earliest part of life such as embryogenesis. With this notion in mind, Medawar reversed the usual idea concerning senescence and the coming of old age. Indeed, it was often thought that old age began with the termination of reproduction, because without reproduction individuals could not make a biological contribution to future generations. To Medawar, however, the cessation of reproduction was merely a *consequence* of the accumulation of senile changes that began in early life [85]. What was thus necessary was to explain the end of reproduction as a result of aging process rather than to account for the start of old age through the termination of reproduction. To conceptualize this process, Medawar adopted Fisher's "reproductive value" in a simplified form under a hypothetical condition suggested by Lotka. Citing Lotka, who postulated an unreal condition in which death occurred only due to accidents without the influence of senescence [86], Medawar suggested a situation in which the birth rate and population size did not change and the number of individuals within an age group decreased at a certain fixed rate through random accidents such as predation or disease rather than aging. In this state, the "reproductive value" became a constant [84].

Medawar's evolutionary theory of aging explained how this hypothetical condition should inevitably lead to the emergence of senescence [87]. He claimed that even in a condition without senescence the number of individuals within an age cohort tended to undergo a steady decrease at a certain rate due to disease or predation. In this situation, an age cohort's reproductive contribution to future generations would continuously decline over time at a fixed rate, because the constant reproductive value made the actual contribution of that cohort depend only on the number of its surviving members. According to Medawar, this state influenced the course of evolution. Whereas the time of favorable genes' expression would increasingly move toward the earlier parts of life, that of unfavorable genes would consistently shift to later life due to the weak force of natural selection at that time caused by the small number of survivors. To put simply, natural selection would make the genes that could lower the organism's chance of survival be expressed only in later life when most of these organisms had already perished and could not contribute to future generations. Since these genes, which might include those for terminating reproductive capacity, could undergo further mutations without being influenced by the force of natural selection, their deleterious phenotypic effects would become stronger during the course of evolution. But in the wild state, these genes could hardly get a chance of expression, since most individuals in the wild would have died at that point of time. However, Medawar argued, the human's civilization and the domestication of animals changed the situation. Most domesticated animals and humans would eventually see the effects in the form of wrinkled skin, decline of mental and physical vigor, and various chronic diseases, because they could survive and become old due to better nutrition, health care, and other artificial factors.

This theory, published in 1946, was a culmination of his conceptual work for the past ten years [88]. The theory clearly incorporated the standpoint of Fisher, Thompson, and others who claimed that the temporal dimension of life was significant and could be quantitatively analyzed in theoretical terms. Medawar also included in his theory the new evolutionary ideas of the Modern Synthesis as well as its major contributors' specific concepts. This made his idea considerably different from August Weismann's older evolutionary theory of aging dependent upon group selection [89]. Moreover, Medawar's deeply-held conviction that the temporal dimension of life could not be sharply separated into two phases, namely, growth and senescence, was thoroughly reflected. In his theoretical scheme, there is no clear distinction between aging and growth, because the force of natural selection that created the genes for senescence was applied throughout the whole lifespan with a gradually decreasing intensity. Medawar's new theory of aging addressed the interrelationship among growth, aging, and evolution in a single conceptual framework.

In the same paper, Medawar suggested a possibility of an experimental study of senescence as well. He proposed that it was feasible to transplant tissues between old and young animals to examine how the living cells responded to a different organismic environment of a distinct age. This experiment could answer many questions like the following.

> How, then, does tissue transplanted from a baby animal to a dotard develop in its "old" environment? Does it rapidly mature and age, or does it remain like a new patch on an old pair of socks? Conversely, what is the fate of tissue grafted from old animals into youngsters [88]?

He called the organisms that could address these questions "time-chimeras," which were made through surgical combination of two body parts of distinct ages.

What was significant was that Medawar never made such "time-chimeras" for the study of aging. In fact, he did not pursue any further research on aging for the remainder of his life, even though his theory played an important role in later developments of the evolutionary study of senescence [90-93]. Interestingly, the creation of "time-chimeras" contributed to a seemingly unrelated work. As we will see, he used time-chimeras in his tissue transplantation experiment that confirmed immunological tolerance. While Medawar did not intend in 1946 this use of his idea, the reorientation of his initial proposal did make a small but important contribution to the experiment on immunological tolerance.

It is not hard to find the reason why the use of the proposed experiment was changed. While staying at the University of Birmingham from 1947 to 1951, he spent most of his time and energy not in aging research but in tissue transplantation, which led him to explore a large number of study subjects regarding immunity and other issues. After accepting Jodrell Professorship in Zoology at University College London in 1951, Medawar accounted for this broader applicability of tissue transplantation in a review paper. According to him, the transplantation of skin could be "used for the study of a wide variety of biological problems," such as the nature of pigmentation, the effect of freezing and drying upon the viability of tissues, and the role of different skin layers in engendering tumors under the influence of certain chemicals [94]. It was also possible to use transplantation for investigating the clinical effect of cortisone, measuring the degree of homozygosity of inbred animals, and examining the behavior of cells in anaerobic environments [95, 96]. Medawar and his team were funded by several supporters for implementing these projects, such as the Medical Research Council, the Department of Surgery at the University of Oxford, and the British Empire Cancer Campaign [97]. The scope of tissue transplantation research, which had begun as a wartime project, was thus substantially expanded, enabling Medawar and his team to become highly productive and versatile researchers.

While pursuing these projects, Medawar, however, did not lose his interest in life's temporal dimensions observable through development and evolution. In 1950, he and Billingham grafted the cornea, the sole epithelium, and other tissues to various different portions of the mammalian body and found that these tissues maintained their original histological specificity even after the change of their location. For Medawar and Billingham, this observation meant that the cellular characteristics were "inherited or 'genetic', and [was] not to be attributed to the physiological differences between the environments" [98]. But Medawar also said that the cellular characteristics were a product of developmental process, although their ultimate cause was the genes. In a paper titled "Problems of Adaptation," Medawar stated that the identity and characteristics of a cell were "'laid on' by development" [99]. Admittedly, he did not propose any detailed theories on how cell differentiation occurred during embryogenesis and development and in what degree the genes, the cytoplasmic hereditary enzymes, and the environments were involved in it. Moreover, he did not mean that a cell's type determined during embryogenesis was flexible. The process of making cellular specificity through development was highly deterministic, because it did not allow any further changes, even in an altered environment. What was important in his statement was that Medawar thought that the formation of cellular characteristics was a process that occurred over *time* during development. Perhaps he already ceased to support cytoplasmic inheritance at that time. Nonetheless, as a scientist deeply interested in the dynamic changes of life during growth, aging, and evolution, he did not like to think about the gene's effect in a static term, without considering its temporal dimensions.

In the same paper, Medawar also discussed the evolutionary dimensions of cellular specificity. He argued that the characteristics of the cornea and the sole epithelium had been established during the long evolutionary process according to the Darwinian force of natural selection [99]. In fact, the case of the sole epithelium was different from that of the cornea. The thick skin of the sole could be imitated through repeated mechanical pressure applied by the environment, while the cornea could never be emulated in such a way. Hence, unlike the case of the cornea, that of the sole might be used as a piece of evidence supporting Lamarckism. Yet as a champion of the Modern Synthesis, Medawar did not hope to vindicate Lamarckism. Medawar argued that it was beneficial for the organism to have these two types of tissues established during developmental process before birth. Since these traits would enhance the chance of survival of the organism in its natural habitat, they were selected during evolutionary process and became an integral part of the mammalian constitution.

During the early 1950s, Medawar wrote other theoretical articles regarding evolution, growth, and aging. In 1950, he published a paper titled, "Transformation of Shape," which discussed various issues concerning the mathematical analysis of development following the methodology of Thompson and Huxley. In this paper, while talking about how continuous changes of shape could be described, he returned to a subject that was important in his early tissue culture research—aging. Since "the mode of growth changes during a lifetime," he said, "functions of different sorts must be used to describe its several phases—first a compound interest function….and later a function describing a die-away of growth rate" [100]. Indeed, while Medawar did not attempt any further discussion of this subject in the paper, his mention of "die-away of growth rate" during development shows his enduring interest in aging in relation to growth. In another paper published in the next year, Medawar expressed his deep respect toward the scientists who provided him with the theoretical resources and broad dynamic perspectives on living organisms. In his chapter on "Zoology" in *Scientific Thought in the Twentieth Century*, Medawar criticized vitalists and holists' "active detestation of mathematical analysis," and cited several scholars—including Lotka, Fisher, Simpson, Wright, Huxley, and Thompson—who stood on the other side [101]. To Medawar, their rigorous mathematical research on growth and evolution established a strong foundation of modern biological investigation.

Another theoretical article published in 1952 dealt with a narrower subject concerning immunological individuality. This paper, titled "A Biological Analysis of Individuality," showed Medawar's growing ideas on the nature of immunological identity that he had been concerned about for years. In 1946, he argued that the formation of individuality was a complex process that had developmental, hereditary, and evolutionary dimensions [77]. In 1952, he excluded any discussion on the genetic or evolutionary aspects of individuality and focused on its developmental side. He claimed that immunological individuality was "a property that comes into being during the course of development" [102].

But even with regard to the developmental dimension, the meaning of individuality was different from that in the past. While Medawar in 1946 had discussed the growth of individuality based on the nonresponse of young animals toward extrinsic agent, his 1952 article had a new resource that had a more profound implication. At the time, Medawar came to read a paper by Ray Owen, which made a contribution to Burnet's conception of his notion of immunological "self"[51]. For Medawar, like Burnet, Owen's observation revealed that developing animals could continue to be unresponsive to extrinsic agents even after the end of their growth phase. Whereas there had already been several cases showing that the embryo and the fetus did not immunologically respond to extrinsic agents, it had still been found that rejection ultimately occurred in all these cases after the end of growth period. In contrast, Owen's research revealed that it was possible for an animal to permanently retain genetically distinct portions that had coexisted with it during development. By incorporating this work of Owen, Medawar changed the meaning of individuality from something that merely grew during developmental periods to what was actively *defined* in these phases.

In fact, Owen's observation was a significant discovery for homograft problem as well. Past researchers and surgeons had known a small number of exceptional instances when homograft rejection did not occur, such as tissue exchange between monozygotic twins, grafting of foreign tissues into the brain or the eye's anterior chamber, or transplantation of skin between two highly inbred animals. To Medawar, Owen's observation was a significant addition to this short list of immunological tolerance and an instance pertaining to his idea on immunological individuality, about which a further experimental study was expected.

Interestingly, Medawar did not mention Erich Traub's papers while citing Owen's article. As I have written, Burnet incorporated both Traub's and Owen's research in making his theory of immunological tolerance. This reflected Burnet's unique perspectives derived from his medical training and subsequent research career in virology, epidemiology, and etiology. To Medawar, who did not share this training and career, only Owen's paper was meaningful. Traub's papers dealt with subjects in which he was not very interested and did not have expertise, such as virology and the "equilibrium" between the host and the parasite. Perhaps Medawar did not even think that these subjects were related to what Owen showed in his paper.

There were other research articles with related implication. As I have shown, Burnet himself along with his colleagues conducted an experiment on immunological tolerance using viruses and red blood cells, although he did not obtain a result that fit with his expectation [55]. A more interesting work was published in 1952 by Jack A. Cannon and William P. Longmire at the University of California, Los Angeles. They arrived at a more successful result using chickens' skin homograft rather than inoculation of viruses and cells as Burnet did. In this experiment, Cannon and Longmire found that the age of the chicken was closely related to the length of homografts' survival time in a new host. While about thirteen percent of the chickens that had received a homograft patch right after hatching retained it by the eight week, only one percent among those that had acquired a homograft from the fourth to the sixth day still kept it in the same week [103]. The younger the host organism was at the time of surgery, the longer the extrinsic transplant could survive on the skin. An older paper cited in this article by Cannon and Longmire also showed an interesting result. In 1929, C. H. Danforth and Frances Foster at Stanford University argued that twenty-nine among one hundred and eighty-eight chickens that had received a graft from a different individual "on the day of hatching or within a few days thereafter" could retain it almost indefinitely [104]. Since twelve among these twenty-nine chickens had obtained a graft from the same strain, the number of surviving homografts from completely unrelated individuals was seventeen, which was quite impressive.

In the early 1950s, Medawar was aware of Burnet's article, but there is no evidence that he read the papers by Cannon, Longmire, Danforth, and Foster. Cannon and Longmire's article came out in 1952 when Medawar was conducting his landmark research that would be published in 1953. Since Medawar's archival collection does not have any correspondence with them, it is unlikely that they exerted any influence upon the implementation of Medawar's experiment. In contrast, Danforth and Foster's older experiments had already been performed in the 1920s, and it is thus possible that Medawar had known of it. Yet Medawar did not cite their works in his crucial papers on tolerance published during the early 1950s. Indeed, the aim and design of Medawar's experiments were very different from theirs. While Danforth and Foster merely tried to show that tissues could survive for a long time in a foreign host when they were transplanted onto it in its early age, Medawar aimed at investigating whether the host could *remember* the structure and pattern of the molecules and cells—some of which could have a foreign origin—within its body during its early developmental phase. Although Medawar did not explicitly discuss the issue of immunological individuality in his papers published during the early 1950s, it was already assumed in the design of his experiment.

The first study under this design was Medawar and his colleagues's experiments using dizygotic twin calves conducted during the early 1950s at Cold Norton Farm in Staffordshire. Following Owen's line of research and cooperating with the Animal Breeding and Genetics Research Organization in Edinburgh, Medawar's team performed their experiments and arrived at a remarkable conclusion. They found that that "all two-egg twins show some degree of tolerance to homografts transplanted from one to the other," and that "thirty-six out of 42 cattle of two-egg twin birth were found to be completely tolerant to skin homograft" [105].

While using dizygotic twin calves like Owen, Medawar's study had a deeper implication for immunology in at least two respects. First, Medawar's experiment suggested evidence that the calves might be able to remember the whole body's pattern of their dizygotic twin brother or sister as a part of their own constitution. Indeed, what was immediately obvious in his experiment was the fact that skin could be exchanged as well as blood between dizygotic twins. But skin was different from blood. It was an *ad hoc* addition to the animal's body, while blood was just descendents from the original cells that had migrated through connected blood vessels. In this sense, Medawar's experiment presented a stronger proof that something that had been exchanged during fetal life could be permanently tolerated. Moreover, it was possible that the skin cell was just one of those that had been shared in early life. Other sorts of cells must have been exchanged as well, and perhaps the whole body's pattern of the dizygotic twin might be remembered by the other calf. Second, Medawar's experiment showed more details and complex aspects of tolerance phenomenon than Owen's. It was found that "the degree of tolerance" among them was "widely variable." While complete tolerance toward their dizygotic twin's skin was found in the thirty-six cattle among the forty-two that had been examined, the six individuals also showed varied degrees of tolerance, measured by the number of days during which the skin patch survived in the host body. Moreover, it was found that the "grafts from one twin to the other may be tolerated although grafts of the reciprocal transplantation are eventually destroyed" [105]. This finding meant that tolerance was a complex phenomenon which might not happen to the two organisms that shared blood in fetal phase in the same mode and manner. Hence, the details of tolerance demanded more systematic investigation using an animal model which was easier to handle, such as the mouse.

In designing his new study, Medawar returned to the issue of the age of experimental organisms. If a skin patch was grafted to an unrelated adult animal, it was invariably rejected due to the immune response of the host. But the above experiments using cows and Owen's observation showed that an entity from an external origin could be tolerated if the host organism was in its embryonic or fetal stage. In fact, the papers by Danforth, Foster, Cannon, and Longmire revealed that the host could be slightly older, since some newly hatched chickens also accepted extraneous tissues. What, then, happened during these early periods of an animal? Unlike Burnet, Medawar was not interested in making a detailed theory on the mechanism of immunity formation during growth phases. But this does not mean that Medawar did not make any theories. As I have shown in this monograph, Medawar proposed many theoretical ideas, although these were more abstract, based primarily on mathematical reasoning. In fact, he read and cited the second edition of Burnet's *Production of Antibodies*, but did not attempt to evaluate or discuss the mechanism proposed by Burnet. He simply mentioned that there might be some "profound theoretical reasons" in this changing immune response of a growing animal [106].

As a conceptual resource guiding his experiments, Medawar's own previous research was more important than Burnet's 1949 theory. In 1945, he already found that young rabbits aged between 2½ and 4½ weeks old did not differ from older rabbits in terms of immune response to homografts [71]. Rather than thinking that age was irrelevant to homograft response, he concluded that the ability to recognize and attack foreign materials had fully developed before the rabbit reached 2½ weeks of age. In fact, other scientists' studies, especially those after James Murphy, did indicate that the critical age of immunity development should be found in earlier periods, namely, the phase of embryogenesis [45]. It is also quite remarkable that Medawar was thinking about "time-chimeras" again. After completing his experiment on the effect of freezing on the viability of cells in 1952, he argued that "one possible approach to the problem of the cause of senescence is to graft tissue from a young animal to its own self when it has grown older" [107]. It was possible to detach tissues from a young animal and to store them in a freezer until the organism became older. Then, the frozen "young" tissues could be thawed and regrafted to their original host to investigate a variety of issues concerning aging.

Medawar and his colleagues' well-known research published in their 1953 paper was initiated from making this time-chimera, although it was a genetic chimera as well. He injected a "suspension of adult tissue cells" of an A-line mouse into six fetuses within the uterus of a CBA mouse. These chimeras between the young CBA and the older A-line mouse grew well except one which died before birth. After these remaining five mice became eight weeks old, they received A-line skin grafts. Remarkably, two out of the five mice showed complete tolerance toward these grafts, while other two mice quickly rejected them. The remaining one "underwent a long-drawn-out 'spontaneous' involution" which resulted in the "complete breakdown shortly after the 91st day" of transplantation [2].

Along with this observation, two interesting additional experiments were simultaneously done. The first, which involved grafting of a third strain's tissue into the chimeras, showed that tolerance was highly specific, by revealing that these grafts were rapidly rejected. The second experiment was about the organs responsible for tolerance. After "fragments of lymph node from normal CBA mice which had been actively immunized against A-line skin" were inserted into the two surviving chimeras, their skin grafts, which had been perfectly integrated into the host body by that time, were ultimately broken down. This result showed that tolerance phenomenon was dependent on the immune cells in the lymph node which *learned* not to respond to a specific group of tissues.

Medawar's success in these experiments that led to the Nobel Prize was indebted to a variety of factors, including his expertise in tissue transplantation, Owen's 1945 paper, and Burnet's *Production of Antibodies*. But Medwar's long concern about the temporal dimensions of the living organism was a crucial contributing factor as well, which could be seen in the following statement.

> The effect of this first presentation of foreign tissue in adult life is to confer 'immunity', that is, to increase the host's resistance to grafts....But if the first presentation of foreign cells takes place in foetal life, it has just the opposite effect: resistance to a graft transplanted on some later occasion, so far from being heightened, is abolished or at least reduced. Over some period of its early life, therefore, the pattern of the host's response to foreign tissue cells is turned completely upside down. In mice....this inversion takes place in the neighborhood of birth, for there is a certain 'null' period thereabouts when the inoculation of foreign tissue confers neither tolerance nor heightened resistance [2].

Medawar and his team actually conducted an experiment to confirm the existence of this "null period." This study was very remarkable, because he intended a systematic research using a large number of mice. Whereas he used only five mice in examining the development of tolerance during the fetal period, total ninety-six newly born mice were used to investigate the null period. When these very young mice were inoculated with foreign tissues and were later challenged with the tissues from the same donor after they became adults, only nine among them revealed tolerance to the extrinsic tissue. A large portion of the remaining mice showed neither tolerance nor immunity. This result implied that the "null period" did exist as a stage in an animal's life and that age was a key factor in the growth of immunological identity and tolerance.

Medawar's interest in the role of age in immunity and tolerance can also be found in his 1956 paper, titled, "Quantitative Studies on Tissue Transplantation Immunity. III. Actively Acquired Tolerance" [108]. This paper shows his mathematical expertise and dynamic perspective very well. He reused the probit transformation techniques to calculate the median survival time (MST) of homografts. The MST was used to make a standard against which the degree of immune response or tolerance could be measured. This paper was also remarkable due to its use of a large number of several distinct research organisms, including rabbits, rats, and chickens. The data from these sets of experiments gave a further support to Medawar's conclusion on tolerance written in the 1953 paper. But perhaps a most significant feature of his 1956 paper is that Medawar showed the result of his in-depth study of age-dependence of tolerance. Indeed, he inoculated with the same foreign cells two groups of mouse fetuses before and after the eighteenth day of conception. While the group that received the foreign cells at an older age showed slightly a higher percentage of mice with initial tolerance, the group that was inoculated at an earlier phase was eventually revealed to have a larger proportion of fetuses with long-term tolerance after the fiftieth day. Considering the difficulty of inoculation into a very young fetus before the eighteenth day of conception, these results clearly showed that it was easier to induce tolerance to external agents in younger organisms.

In the same paper, Medawar and his team also conducted another set of experiments on the "null period," reconfirming the previous conclusion. In the case of mice, it was the immediate postnatal phase that tolerance was changed into immune response. Citing Cannon and Longmire's experiments as well, Medwar and his colleagues claimed that these and other experiments clearly showed "the progressive decay, with increasing age, of the power of an antigenic stimulus to confer tolerance" [108].

This statement of Medawar will remind many readers of his reference to Minot's thesis in his 1941 paper on tissue culture. While Medawar's research subject in 1956 was very different from what he studied in 1941, his view of aging as a phenomenon that proceeded even in the earliest part of life could still be seen in the above remark. In a deeper sense, Medawar found what he wanted to study, namely, a process that occurred throughout an animal's entire lifespan. Like aging and tissue's survivability outside of the body, the ability to incorporate extrinsic agents underwent rapid decline in early life.

Chapter 4

CONCLUSION

Both Burnet and Medawar contributed to the development of immunology, while their approaches and perspectives were highly different. Burnet conceived his theory of "self" and "tolerance" through his study of medical microbiology, etiology, and epidemiology, which taught him the importance of ecological balance between the host and the pathogen as well as the critical significance of the host's age in disease causation. In this work, I also showed that cytoplasmic inheritance theories were another key factor that facilitated Burnet's theorization in immunology. In contrast, Medawar formulated his ideas on immunological "individuality" and succeeded in conducting an experiment on "acquired immune tolerance" through his expertise in tissue transplantation and his theoretical works on aging, growth, and evolution. While both scientists regarded temporal and dynamic dimensions of living organisms as important, the pathways through which they developed their ideas of "self" and "tolerance" were highly distinct.

Furthermore, a more careful look at the two scientists' studies reveals that even within their works several different traditions of research were actively synthesized. In the case of Burnet, a number of medical fields, especially virology, epidemiology, and etiology, were combined with the concepts in the non-medical life sciences, namely, cytoplasmic inheritance theories. Likewise, Medawar synthesized his works on aging, growth, and evolution with his tissue transplantation study. These syntheses show that the conceptualization of immunological "self" and the experimental induction of "tolerance" were a result of a hybridization of various distinct lines of investigation within medical and biological subdisciplines.

Indeed, hybridization of research traditions, which is often not planned or anticipated, is not uncommon in the history of science. According to philosopher and historian Rheinberger, the course of scientific research is often far from coherent and organized. Through his historical study of *in vitro* protein synthesis, he claimed that there are instances of unpredictable changes of study directions and accidental merger of two or more distinct lines of research at a single point. Rheinberger used his concept of "conjuncture" to account for these instances. As his case study of protein synthesis showed, several seemingly unrelated research projects could accidentally meet at a single place of conjuncture and be represented in a very novel and unexpected way. He argues that the making of such conjunctures is a feature of productive scientific research programs or "experimental systems."

While Rheinberger has proposed this concept in his grand philosophical attack against the modernist epistemology of science, my aim in this monograph is more modest and historically more specific. I have shown that the relationship between Burnet and Medawar reveals how accidental encounters among research programs and study fields were possible during the mid-twentieth century in Australia and Britain. Such encounters brought about a productive hybridization, as can be seen in the scientific career of the two investigators. As we know well, the hybridization of Burnet's and Medawar's research brought about a remarkable change in immunology.

REFERENCES

[1] Burnet FM, Fenner F. The production of antibodies. 2nd ed. Melbourne: Macmillan; 1949.
[2] Billingham RE, Brent L, Medawar PB. "Actively acquired tolerance" of foreign cells. *Nature* 1953;172:603-6.
[3] Nossal GJV. Some landmarks in Australian immunology. *Immunol. Cell Biol.* 1991;69:327-35.
[4] Martini A, Burgio GR. Tolerance and auto-immunity: 50 years after Burnet. *Eur. J. Pediatr.* 1999;158:769-75.
[5] Mackay IR. The "Burnet era" of immunology: origins and influence. *Immunol. Cell Biol.* 1991;69:301-5.
[6] Sexton C. Seeds of time: the life of Sir Macfarlane Burnet. Oxford: Oxford University Press; 1991.
[7] Tauber AI, Podolsky SH. Frank Macfarlane Burnet and the immune self. *J. Hist. Biol.* 1994;27:531-73.
[8] Tauber AI. The immune self: theory of metaphor? Cambridge: Cambridge University Press; 1994.
[9] Crist E, Tauber AI. Selfhood, immunity, and the biological imagination: the thought of Frank Macfarlane Burnet. *Biol. Philos.* 2000;15:509-33.
[10] Silverstein AM. A history of immunology. San Diego: Academic Publishers; 1989.
[11] Löwy I. The strength of loose concepts—boundary concepts, federative strategies and disciplinary growth: the case of immunology. *Hist. Sci.* 1992;30:371-96.
[12] Park HW. Germs, hosts, and the origin of Frank Macfarlane Burnet's concept of "self" and "tolerance," 1936-1949. *J. Hist. Med. All Sci.* 2006;61:492-534.

[13] Mitchison NA. Peter Brian Medawar, 28 February 1951-2 October 1987. Biographical memoirs of fellows of the Royal Society. 1990;35:283-301.
[14] Mitchison NA. Sir Peter Medawar (1915-1987). *Nature* 1987;330:112
[15] Gowans JL. Peter Medawar: his life and work. *Immunol. Lett.* 1989;21:5-8.
[16] Hamilton D. Peter Medawar and clinical transplantation. *Immunol. Lett.* 1989;21:9-13.
[17] Simpson E. Reminiscence of Sir Peter Medawar: in hope of antigen-specific transplantation tolerance. *Am. J. Transplant.* 2004;4:1937-40.
[18] The Nobel Chronicles. *Lancet* 1999;353:2253.
[19] Möller G. Sir Peter Medawar. *Immunol. Rev.* 1987;100:9-10.
[20] Tanner J. Sir Peter Medawar, 1915-1987. *Ann. Hum. Biol.* 1988;15:89.
[21] Burnet FM. Changing patterns: an atypical autobiography. Melbourne: William Heinemann; 1968.
[22] Shapin S, Schaffer S. Leviathan and the air-pump: Hobbes, Boyle, and the experimental life. Princeton: Princeton University Press; 1985.
[23] Medawar PB. Memoir of a thinking radish: an autobiography. Oxford: Oxford University Press; 1988.
[24] Rheinberger HJ. Towards a history of epistemic things: synthesizing proteins in the test tube. Stanford: Stanford University Press; 1997.
[25] Fenner F. The John Murtaph Macrossan lecture: Sir Macfarlane Burnet scientist and thinker. St. Lucia: University of Queensland Press; 1988.
[26] Amsterdamska O. Medical and biological constraints: early research on variation in bacteriology. *Soc. Stud. Sci.* 1987;17:657-87.
[27] Ledingham, JCG, Arkwright JA. The carrier problem in infectious diseases. London, Edward Arnold; 1912.
[28] Carter, KC. The rise of causal concepts of disease: case histories. Aldershot: Ashgate; 2003.
[29] Worboys M. Spreading germs: disease theories and medical practices in Britain, 1865-1900. Cambridge: Cambridge University Press; 2000.
[30] Burnet FM. Lysogenicity as a normal function of certain salmonella strains. *J. Pathol. Bacteriol.* 1932;35:851-63.
[31] Burnet FM. Recent work on the biological nature of bacteriophages. *Trans. R. Soc. Trop. Med. Hyg.* 1933;26:409-16.
[32] Burnet FM, Williams SW. Herpes simplex: a new point of view. *Med. J. Aust.* 1939;1:637-42.
[33] Burnet FM. The rickettsial disease in Australia. *Med. J. Aust.* 1942;2:129-34.

[34] Burnet FM. Biological aspects of infectious disease. Cambridge: Cambridge University Press; 1940.
[35] Burnet FM, Freeman M. Experimental studies on the virus of "Q" fever. *Med. J. Aust.* 1937;2:299-305.
[36] Burnet FM. The biological approach to infectious disease. *Med. J. Aust.* 1941;2:607-12.
[37] Wells HG, Huxley JS, Wells GP. The science of life: a summary of contemporary knowledge about life and its possibilities. London: Amalgamated Press; 1929.
[38] Mendelsohn JA. From eradication to equilibrium: how epidemics became complex after World War I. In: Lawrence C, Weisz G, editors. Greater than the parts: holism in biomedicine, 1920-1950. New York: Oxford University Press; 1998. p. 303-31.
[39] Mendelsohn JA. Medicine and the making of bodily inequality in twentieth century Europe. In: Gaudillière GP, Löwy I, editors. Heredity and infection: the history of disease transmission. London: Routledge; 2001. p. 21-79.
[40] Kunitz SJ. Explanations and ideologies of mortality patterns. *Popul. Dev. Rev.* 1987;13:379-408.
[41] Löwy I. On guinea pigs, dogs and men: anaphylaxis and the study of biological individuality, 1902-1939. *Stud. Hist. Phil. Biol. Biomed. Sci.* 2003;34:399-423.
[42] Kroker K. Immunity and its other: the anaphylactic selves of Charles Richet. *Stud. Hist. Phil. Biol. Biomed. Sci.* 1999;30:273-96.
[43] Parnes O. Troubles from within: allergy, autoimmunity, and pathology in the first half of the twentieth century. *Stud. Hist. Phil. Biol. Biomed. Sci.* 2003;34:425-54.
[44] Burnet FM, Freeman M, Jackson AV, Lush D. The production of antibodies: a review and a theoretical discussion. 1st ed. Melbourne: Macmillan; 1941.
[45] Murphy JB. Transplantability of tissues to the embryo of foreign species: its bearing on questions of tissue specificity and tumor immunity. *J. Exp. Med.* 1913;17:482-92.
[46] Smith T, Kilborne FL. Investigations into the nature, causation, and prevention of Texas or Southern cattle fever. Washington: Government Printing Office; 1893.
[47] Burnet FM. The epidemiology of poliomyelitis, with special reference to the Victorian epidemic of 1397-38. *Med. J. Aust.* 1940;1:325-36.

[48] Burnet FM. Antibody production in the light of recent genetic theory. *Aust. J. Sci.* 1946;8:143-6.
[49] Burnet FM. The basis of allergic disease. *Med. J. Aust.* 1948;1:29-35.
[50] Sapp J. Beyond the gene: cytoplasmic inheritance and the struggle for authority in genetics Oxford: Oxford University Press; 1987.
[51] Owen RD. Immunogenetic consequences of vascular anastomoses between bovine twins. *Science.* 1945;102:400-1.
[52] Traub E. The epidemiology of lymphocytic choriomeningitis in white mice. *J. Exp. Med.* 1936;64:183-200.
[53] Traub E. Factors influencing the persistence of choriomeningitis virus in the blood of mice after clinical recovery. *J. Exp. Med.* 1938;68:229-50.
[54] Traub E. Epidemiology of lymphocytic choriomeningitis in a mouse stock observed for four years. *J. Exp. Med.* 1939;69:801-17.
[55] Burnet FM, Stone JD, Edney M. The failure of antibody production in the chick embryo. *Aust. J. Exp. Biol. Med. Sci.* 1950;28:291-8.
[56] Jerne NK. The natural-selection theory of antibody formation. *Proc. Nat. Acad. Sci. U.S.A.* 1955;41:849-57.
[57] Burnet FM. A modification of Jerne's theory of antibody production using the concept of clonal selection. *Aust. J. Sci.* 1957;20:67-9.
[58] Thompson DW. On growth and form. Cambridge: Cambridge University Press; 1917.
[59] Medawar PB. Size, shape, and age. In: Clark WELG, Medawar PB, editors. Essays on growth and form presented to D'Arcy Wentworth Thompson. Oxford: Clarendon; 1945. p. 157-87.
[60] Medawar PB. The shape of the human being as a function of time. *Proc. Roy. Soc. B-Biol. Sci.* 1944;132:133-41.
[61] Morrell J. Science at Oxford, 1914-1939: transforming an arts university. Oxford: Oxford University Press; 1997.
[62] Medawar PB. Oxford zoology. *Biol.* 1944;Autumn:1-4.
[63] Medawar PB. A factor inhibiting the growth of mesenchyme. *Q. J. Exp. Physiol.* 1937;27:147-60.
[64] Medawar PB. The growth, growth energy, and ageing of the chicken's heart. *Proc. Roy. Soc. B-Biol. Sci.* 1940;129:332-55.
[65] Minot CS. The problem of age, growth, and death: a study of cytomorphosis. New York: Putnam; 1908.
[66] Medawar PB. The 'laws' of biological growth. *Nature.* 1941;148:772-4.
[67] Medawar PB. The rate of penetration of fixatives. *J. Roy Microsc. Soc.* 1941;60:46-57.

[68] Jacoby E, Medawar PB, Willmer EN. The toxicity of sulphonamide drugs to cells in vitro. *Brit. Med. J.* 1941;2:149-53.
[69] Gibson T, Medawar PB. The fate of skin homograft in man. *J. Anat.* 1943;77:299-310.
[70] Medawar PB. Notes on the problem of skin homografts. *Bull. War Med.* 1943;4:1-4.
[71] Medawar PB. A second study of the behavior and fate of skin homograft in rabbits. *J. Anat.* 1945;79:157-77.
[72] Medawar PB. The behavior and fate of skin autografts and skin homografts in rabbits. *J. Anat.* 1944;78:176-99.
[73] Gutmann E, Guttmann L, Medawar PB, Young JZ. The rate of regeneration of nerve. *J. Exp. Biol.* 1942;19:14-44.
[74] Medawar PB. Biological aspects of the repair process. *Brit. Med. Bull.* 1945;3:70-3.
[75] Billingham RE, Medawar PB. The 'cytogenetics' of black and white guinea.pig skin. *Nature.* 1947;159:115-7.
[76] Medawar PB. Cellular inheritance and transformation. *Biol. Rev.* 1947;22:360-89.
[77] Medawar PB. The theory of the differences between individuals. The substance of a lecture given to the Oxford summer school of the British Social Hygiene Council. 1946. Peter Brian Medawar Papers, Box 36, Folder E.23, Wellcome Library, London, England.
[78] Medawar PB. Asymmetry of larval Amphioxus. *Nature.* 1951;167:852-3.
[79] Huxley J. Evolution: the modern synthesis. New York: Harpers; 1942.
[80] Haldane JBS. The time of action of genes, and its bearings on some evolutionary problems. *Am. Nat.* 1932;66:5-24.
[81] Ford EB, Huxley J. Genetic rate-factors in Gammarus. *Roux. Arch. Dev. Biol.* 1929;117:67-79.
[82] Simpson GG. Tempo and mode in evolution. New York: Columbia University Press; 1944.
[83] Fisher RA. Genetical theory of natural selection. Oxford: Oxford University Press; 1930.
[84] Medawar PB. Demography: notes. Undated. Peter Brian Medawar Papers, Box 17, Folder C.26, Wellcome Library, London, England.
[85] Medawar PB. An unsolved problem of biology: an inaugural lecture delivered at University College London, 6 December 1951. London: Lewis; 1952.

[86] Lotka AJ. Elements of physical biology. Baltimore: Williams and Wilkins; 1925.
[87] Medawar PB. Special case. Undated. Peter Brian Medawar Papers, Box 17, Folder C.23, Wellcome Library, London, England.
[88] Medawar PB. Old age and natural death. *Mod. Quart.* 1946;2:30-49.
[89] Weismann A. Essays upon heredity and kindred biological problems. Poulton, EB, Schönland S, Shipley, AE, editors. Oxford: Clarendon; 1889.
[90] Charlesworth B. Fisher, Medawar, Hamilton, and the evolution of aging. *Genetics.* 2000;156:927-31.
[91] Gavrilov LA, Gavrilova NS. Evolutionary theories of aging and longevity. *Sci. World J.* 2002;2:339-56.
[92] Holliday R. The evolution of human longevity. *Perspect. Biol. Med.* 1996;40:100-7.
[93] Rose MR, Graves JL. What evolutionary biology can do for gerontology. *J. Gerontol. A-Biol.* 1989;44:B27-9.
[94] Billingham RE, Medawar PB. The technique of free skin grafting in mammals. *J. Exp. Biol.* 1951;28:385-402.
[95] Billingham RE, Krohn PL, Medawar PB. Effect of cortisone on survival of skin homografts in rabbits. *Brit. Med. J.* 1951;1:1157-63.
[96] Medawar PB. The behaviour of mammalian skin epithelium under strictly anaerobic conditions. *Q. J. Microsc. Sci.* 1947;88:27-37.
[97] Billingham RE, Medawar PB. Pigment spread in mammalian skin: serial propagation and immunity reactions. *Heredity.* 1950;4:141-64.
[98] Billingham RE, Medawar PB. A note on the specificity of the corneal epithelium. *J. Anat.* 1950;84:50-7.
[99] Medawar PB. Problems of adaptation. In: Johnson ML, Abercrombie M, editors. New Biology. Vol. 11. London: Penguin; 1951. p. 10-26.
[100] Medawar PB. Transformation of shape. *Proc. Roy. Soc. B-Biol. Sci.* 1950;137:474-9.
[101] Medawar PB. Zoology. In: Heath AE, editor. Scientific thought in the twentieth century London: Watts; 1951. p. 163-89.
[102] Medawar PB. A biological analysis of individuality. *Am. Sci.* 1952;40:632-9.
[103] Cannon JA, Longmire WP. Studies of successful skin homografts in the chicken. *Ann. Surg.* 1952;135:60-8.
[104] Danforth CH, Foster F. Skin transplantation as a means of studying genetic and endocrine factors in the fowl. *J. Exp. Zool.* 1929;52:443-70.

[105] Billingham RE, Lampkin GH, Medawar PB, Williams HL. Tolerance to homografts, twin diagnosis, and the freemartin condition in cattle. *Heredity.* 1952;6:201-12.
[106] Anderson D, Billingham RE, Lampkin GH, Medawar PB. The use of skin grafting to distinguish between monozygotic and dizygotic twins in cattle. *Heredity.* 1951;5:379-97.
[107] Billingham RE, Medawar PB. The freezing, drying and storage of mammalian skin. *J. Exp. Biol.* 1952;29:454-68.
[108] Billingham RE, Brent L, Medawar PB. Quantitative study on tissue transplantation immunity. III. Actively acquired tolerance. *Phil. Trans. Roy. Soc. B-Biol. Sci.* 1956;239:357-414.

INDEX

A

acceleration, 36
accidental, x, 62
accidents, 47
achievement, ix, 2
acquired immunity, 38, 39
adaptation, 17, 18, 29, 68
adaptive enzyme, 16, 24, 28
adult, 17, 21, 25, 40, 45, 56, 57, 58
adults, 17, 19, 20, 21, 27, 46, 58
age, ix, 4, 8, 18, 19, 20, 21, 24, 27, 35, 36, 40, 41, 47, 48, 49, 55, 56, 57, 59, 61, 66, 68
ageing, 34, 66
agent, 8, 14, 18, 25, 26, 29, 41, 53
agents, 17, 21, 22, 27, 30, 41, 44, 45, 53, 59
aging, x, 4, 33, 36, 43, 45, 47, 48, 49, 50, 51, 52, 57, 59, 61, 68
aging process, 36, 47
air, 8, 64
allergy, 65
alternative, 3
anaerobic, 50, 68
anaphylaxis, 14, 21, 65
anastomoses, 66
anastomosis, 24

animals, 17, 18, 22, 24, 27, 30, 34, 38, 44, 45, 48, 49, 50, 53, 54
Antibodies, 1, 15, 16, 17, 25, 27, 57, 58
antibody, 15, 16, 17, 18, 23, 30, 44, 66
antigen, 14, 15, 16, 29, 38, 44, 64
argument, 10, 23, 31, 47
assumptions, 7
Australia, ix, 7, 8, 62, 64
authority, 66
autografts, 67
autoimmunity, 65
awareness, 15
axon, 40

B

babies, 19
bacillus, 14
bacteria, 10, 11, 12, 14, 21, 24, 26
bacterial, 15, 27, 30
bacterial infection, 15
bacteriophage, 10
bacteriophages, 7, 9, 64
barrier, 26
beer, 2
behavior, 24, 26, 27, 50, 67
benign, 9
birds, 45
birth, 5, 47, 52, 56, 57, 58
birth rate, 47

births, 30
blood, 24, 26, 30, 38, 44, 56, 66
blood group, 44
blood transfusion, 38
blood vessels, 56
bloodstream, 16, 28
borrowing, 16
bovine, 66
brain, 14, 20, 54
Brazil, 33
breakdown, 39, 58
Britain, ix, 46, 62, 64

C

calf, 56
carrier, 8, 10, 12, 64
case study, 62
cattle, 19, 21, 24, 30, 56, 65, 69
causation, 8, 13, 15, 18, 20, 61, 65
cell, 16, 22, 23, 28, 29, 36, 40, 41, 42, 51, 56
cell differentiation, 22, 42, 51
Cellulose, ii
chemicals, 50
chicken, 30, 35, 36, 55, 66, 68
chickens, 17, 55, 57, 59
children, 9, 18, 19, 20, 21, 27
chimera, 57
choriomeningitis, 25, 26, 66
chronic disease, 48
chronic diseases, 48
circulation, 24
classical, 26, 44
cohort, 48
collaboration, 4
Columbia, 67
Columbia University, 67
communication, 2, 3
community, 34
complement, 42
components, 24
concentration, 35
conception, 23, 25, 53, 59
conceptualization, 5, 24, 41, 43, 61

Congress, v
constraints, 64
construction, 30, 34
conviction, 9, 49
cornea, 17, 51, 52
corneal epithelium, 68
cows, 24, 56
critical period, 41
culture, 18, 22, 24, 36, 47, 52, 59
Cyanobacteria, ii
cytogenetics, 67
cytoplasm, 22, 23, 28, 41, 43
cytoplasmic inheritance, 4, 22, 23, 28, 41, 42, 51, 61, 66

D

daughter cells, 16, 23
death, 9, 14, 20, 21, 47, 66, 68
decay, 59
definition, 18
deformation, 37
destruction, 12
developmental process, 13, 23, 44, 46, 51, 52
differentiation, 23, 42, 44, 51
diphtheria, 9
disaster, 20
diseases, 21
dizygotic, 24, 55, 56, 69
dizygotic twins, 24, 56, 69
doctors, 7, 15
dogs, 65
domestication, 48
donor, 1, 39, 58
donors, 40
dosage, 39
drugs, 37, 67
drying, 50, 69
duplication, 35

E

ecological, ix, 9, 12, 13, 28, 61

ecologists, 12
educational background, 5
egg, 24, 56
embryo, 22, 24, 28, 29, 30, 35, 41, 46, 53, 65, 66
embryogenesis, ix, 22, 24, 28, 29, 41, 42, 45, 46, 47, 51, 57
embryos, 17, 18, 22, 27, 29
employment, 41, 43
endocrine, 68
endothelial cell, 16, 24
endothelial cells, 16, 24
energy, 35, 50, 66
England, 2, 7, 8, 31, 67, 68
environment, 4, 9, 10, 19, 46, 49, 51, 52
environmental factors, 23
enzymes, 23, 28, 51
epidemic, 65
epidemics, 13, 65
epidemiology, 4, 11, 26, 45, 54, 61, 65, 66
epistemology, 62
epithelium, 51, 52, 68
equilibrium, 10, 54, 65
etiology, 11, 15, 54, 61
Europe, 65
evolution, 11, 13, 20, 21, 33, 43, 44, 45, 46, 48, 49, 51, 52, 61, 67, 68
evolutionary process, 10, 52
exercise, 10
expertise, ix, 4, 43, 54, 58, 59, 61
eye, 54

F

failure, 30, 66
February, 64
fetal, ix, 1, 4, 24, 25, 26, 27, 28, 29, 42, 45, 46, 56, 58
fetus, 1, 22, 29, 53, 59
fetuses, 25, 27, 57, 59
fever, 11, 14, 19, 21, 65
fiber, 40
fixed rate, 48
flare, 10

focusing, 14
food, 12
Ford, 34, 46, 47, 67
foreign organisms, 29
fowl, 68
freezing, 50, 57, 69

G

gender, 8
gene, 52, 66
genes, 13, 22, 38, 42, 44, 46, 47, 48, 49, 51, 67
genetics, x, 66
gerontology, 68
graduate education, 8
grafting, x, 39, 54, 58, 68, 69
grafts, 56, 57, 58
groups, 11, 21, 22, 39, 59
growth, 1, 4, 20, 23, 30, 33, 35, 36, 41, 43, 45, 49, 51, 52, 53, 57, 59, 61, 63, 66
growth rate, 35, 36, 52

H

habitat, 9, 14, 52
harm, 9, 15, 26
health, 19, 49
health care, 49
heart, 35, 66
height, 37
heredity, 43, 68
histological, 51
holism, 65
homozygosity, 50
hospitals, 37
host, ix, 1, 8, 9, 10, 11, 12, 13, 14, 15, 16, 17, 18, 19, 20, 21, 22, 24, 25, 26, 27, 28, 29, 38, 45, 54, 55, 56, 57, 58, 61
human, 9, 17, 19, 20, 27, 30, 36, 48, 66, 68
humans, 10, 11, 19, 21, 29, 36, 48

hunting, 21
hybridization, 61, 62
hygiene, 19
hypothesis, 3, 23, 30
hypothetico-deductive, x, 2, 4

I

identity, 4, 13, 43, 51, 53, 59
imagination, 63
immune cells, 23, 58
immune reaction, 16, 38
immune response, 14, 18, 21, 22, 24, 25, 29, 44, 56, 57, 59
immune system, 8, 15, 17, 18, 21, 30
immunity, 9, 13, 15, 16, 19, 38, 50, 57, 58, 59, 63, 65, 68, 69
immunological, ix, 1, 4, 5, 9, 15, 16, 21, 23, 26, 28, 30, 31, 36, 43, 44, 50, 53, 54, 55, 59, 61
immunologist, 10
immunology, ix, x, 1, 2, 5, 15, 18, 24, 30, 39, 56, 61, 62, 63
implementation, 55
in vitro, 62, 67
incidence, 18, 20, 21, 27
incompatibility, 44
incubation, 44
individuality, 13, 43, 44, 45, 53, 54, 55, 61, 65, 68
induction, 5, 61
inequality, 65
infants, 19, 21, 22, 27
infection, ix, 8, 10, 13, 15, 20, 21, 26, 38, 45, 65
infections, 20, 27
infectious, ix, 2, 4, 7, 8, 9, 10, 11, 12, 14, 17, 18, 20, 21, 22, 27, 29, 45, 64, 65
infectious disease, ix, 2, 4, 7, 8, 9, 10, 11, 12, 14, 18, 20, 21, 22, 27, 29, 45, 64, 65
infectious diseases, 7, 9, 14, 20, 22, 29, 64
infertile, 24
influenza, 19, 20, 27, 30

inheritance, 22, 23, 41, 42, 67
inherited, 16, 23, 28, 42, 51
inhibitory, 35
inhibitory effect, 35
initiation, 3, 19
injuries, 21
injury, v, 41
inoculation, 29, 55, 58, 59
integrity, 13
interaction, 2, 3, 11, 13
interactions, x, 2, 4, 23
interrelations, 33
inversion, 58
Investigations, 65
involution, 58

L

Lamarckism, 52
language, 45
larval, 67
later life, 48
law, 45, 46
laws, 66
lice, 11
life course, 46
life sciences, 61
lifespan, 49, 59
lifetime, 52
limitations, 16
linear, 21
linguistic, 1
location, 2, 9, 23, 37, 51
London, 2, 7, 15, 50, 64, 65, 67, 68
longevity, 68
Los Angeles, 54
lymph, 58
lymph node, 58

M

magnetic, v
malaria, 11
malt extract, 34

mammals, 68
mathematics, 38, 40
median, 59
melanogenesis, 42
men, 65
meningitis, 14
mesenchyme, 66
metaphor, 63
mice, 25, 26, 34, 37, 57, 58, 59, 66
microbes, 7, 10, 11, 21, 22, 26, 44, 45
Microbes, vii, 7
microbial, 8, 10, 26, 38
migration, 42
misleading, 3
molecules, 17, 28, 55
monozygotic twins, 54
morphology, 33
mortality, 20, 21, 27, 40, 65
mortality rate, 20
mouse, 1, 56, 57, 59, 66
movement, 14
MRSA, ii
multiple births, 30
mutant, 20
mutation, 46
mutations, 46, 48

N

nationality, 2
natural, 9, 10, 12, 14, 20, 26, 29, 30, 33, 38, 46, 47, 48, 49, 52, 66, 67, 68
natural habitats, 10, 26
natural selection, 30, 34, 46, 47, 48, 49, 52, 67
nerve, 40, 67
nerves, 40
network, 34
New York, iii, vi, 65, 66, 67
Nobel Prize, ix, 1, 3, 5, 58
normal, 9, 40, 58, 64
normal curve, 40
nuclear, 13, 23, 42, 44
nucleus, 22, 42
nutrition, 19, 49

O

observations, 25, 27
old age, 41, 47
organelle, 22
organism, ix, 1, 12, 13, 16, 17, 18, 20, 23, 36, 38, 40, 41, 43, 45, 46, 48, 52, 55, 56, 57, 58
orientation, 15, 43

P

paradoxical, 36
paralysis, 20
parasite, 10, 11, 17, 26, 45, 54
parasites, 15
parents, 19
Parnes, 14, 65
passive, 8
pathogenic, 11, 14, 19, 21
pathogens, 13, 27
pathology, 65
pathways, ix, 61
patients, x, 8, 14, 37
peripheral nerve, 37, 40
phenotypic, 48
philosophers, 13
philosophical, 62
philosophy, 28
phylogeny, 46
physical biology, 68
physiological, 51
physiology, x, 34
pig, 42, 67
pigs, 65
polio, 19, 20
poliovirus, 19
population, 47
population size, 47
postpartum, 14
power, 41, 59
predators, 29
prediction, ix, 1, 3
pressure, 52

prevention, 65
probability, 40
production, 15, 30, 38, 63, 65, 66
proliferation, 11, 13, 19, 23, 34, 41, 42
propagation, 68
protection, 45
protein, 62
protein synthesis, 62
proteins, 64
protozoa, 19
psittacosis, 10, 20
public, 19
public health, 19

R

race, 18
random, 46, 47, 48
range, 29
rat, 11
rats, 11, 59
reactivity, 16
reading, 3, 11, 19, 34
reasoning, 57
recollection, 37
recovery, 66
red blood cell, 26, 30, 54
red blood cells, 26, 30, 54
regeneration, 40, 41, 67
regular, 22
rejection, 38, 39, 40, 44, 53, 54
relationship, ix, 3, 4, 11, 12, 13, 17, 19, 21, 33, 35, 45, 46, 62
repair, 41, 67
reproduction, 47
research design, 38
residential, 19
resistance, 17, 41, 58
resources, 53
Royal Society, 34, 64
Russian, 13

S

salmonella, 64
Salmonella, 7
school, 67
scientific community, 34
scientific method, 38
scientific understanding, 36
Self, 28
senescence, 35, 36, 47, 48, 49, 50, 57
senile, 36, 47
series, 25, 35, 37
services, v
sex, 18
shape, 17, 28, 29, 41, 52, 66, 68
skin, x, 9, 27, 37, 39, 40, 41, 42, 43, 45, 48, 50, 52, 54, 55, 56, 57, 58, 67, 68, 69
skin grafting, x, 68, 69
social network, 34
somatic cell, 23, 42
somatic cells, 42
species, 45, 46, 65
specificity, 13, 44, 45, 51, 52, 65, 68
speed, 36
spinal cord, 20
stages, 25, 27, 28, 36
Staphylococcus, ii, 9, 18
stimulus, 59
stock, 66
storage, 69
strain, 1, 9, 18, 20, 55, 58
strains, 19, 64
strategies, 63
strength, 63
stress, 42, 43
sulfonamide, 37
summer, 67
sunlight, 10
surgeons, 44, 54
surgery, 55
Surgery, 51
surgical, 50
survivability, 59

survival, 11, 13, 19, 21, 22, 38, 44, 48, 52, 55, 59, 68
surviving, 39, 48, 55, 58
survivors, 18, 48
susceptibility, 35
symbiosis, 10, 12
symptom, 36
symptoms, 8, 10, 14, 18
synthesis, 62, 67

T

temporal, 23, 45, 49, 51, 58, 61
Texas, 19, 21, 65
thinking, 8, 9, 15, 57, 64
throat, 14
ticks, 11
tissue, ix, 1, 2, 4, 17, 22, 26, 34, 35, 36, 39, 40, 41, 43, 44, 45, 47, 49, 50, 52, 54, 57, 58, 59, 61, 65, 69
tolerance, ix, x, 3, 4, 5, 9, 12, 15, 17, 25, 29, 30, 31, 36, 40, 43, 50, 54, 55, 56, 57, 58, 59, 61, 63, 64, 69
toxicity, 37, 67
toxins, 27
training, 2, 4, 7, 26, 31, 54
traits, 52
transformation, 42, 59, 67
transformations, 23
transmission, 65
transplant, 44, 49, 55
transplantation, ix, 1, 2, 4, 22, 26, 34, 38, 40, 41, 43, 45, 50, 54, 56, 58, 61, 64, 68, 69
tuberculosis, 14, 19, 20
tumor, 17, 65
tumors, 50
twins, 56, 66
typhus, 27

U

undergraduate, 33
undergraduate education, 33
uterus, 14, 25, 57

V

vaccination, 9
vaccine, 9
variability, 7
variables, 37
variation, 19, 20, 21, 64
vertebrates, 45
vessels, 56
violent, 17, 30
virological, 12, 45
virology, 4, 45, 54, 61
virulence, 13
virus, 10, 19, 20, 25, 26, 27, 30, 65, 66
viruses, 4, 11, 18, 21, 22, 24, 26, 30, 54

W

war, 38
warfare, 37
Wisconsin, 24
World War, x, 37, 65
World War I, x, 37, 65
World War II, x, 37
writing, 11, 37

Y

yellow fever, 11, 19, 20
young adults, 19, 21, 27

Z

zoology, 33, 66